THE HIDDEN PROTOCOL

REVOLUTIONIZING HOMOEOPATHY: A DATA-DRIVEN APPROACH TO HEALING

DR P NIDHEESH MD(HOM)
DR P RADHAKRISHNAN

"To the pioneers of scientific thought in homoeopathy,
To the practitioners who aspire to standardize and revolutionize patient care,
And to the relentless pursuit of precision in curing the incurable—
This work is dedicated to advancing homoeopathy as a science,
bridging tradition with innovation,
and inspiring a new era of evidence-based healing."

Contents

Contents

Important

● vii ●

MAIL THE INVOICE YOU RECEIVED DURING PURCHASE TO

homoeoschool@gmail.com

To get Access to the Hidden Protocol Software Free for 1 Year.

For Any Queries WhatsApp or Call +91 9072141312

Foreword

As a homoeopath practicing since 1976, I have witnessed the evolution of our field—its triumphs, its challenges, and its untapped potential. Over decades of treating cases of utmost complexity, including a life-altering case of cancer at the age of 24, I have come to realize the immense power of homoeopathy when coupled with precision and unwavering dedication.

This book represents a bold step forward in homoeopathy. It is a testament to the scientific rigor and innovation that this field deserves—a framework designed to transform how we approach patient care. The health scoring and curability assessment introduced in this work are not just concepts but tools that redefine how we perceive, diagnose, and treat our patients. They bridge the gap between art and science, providing clarity and direction in even the most challenging cases.

For practitioners and visionaries alike, this book serves as a beacon of progress. It represents a commitment to advancing homoeopathy as a modern, evidence-based science while preserving its rich tradition. It is a call to action for all who believe in the potential of this great system of medicine.

I commend this effort and its contributions to our field. It is my hope that this work inspires a new generation of practitioners to push the boundaries of what is possible, embracing innovation while holding steadfast to the principles of homoeopathy.

With pride and unwavering belief,
Dr. P. Radhakrishnan
Retired Chief Medical Officer

Preface

It is with immense pride that I present this work, an endeavour that marks a significant step forward in the field of homoeopathy. This book is more than a guide—it is a testament to the transformative power of structured thinking and scientific rigour in patient care. Recognized and copyrighted under the Government of India, this achievement underscores the value and originality of the concepts presented within these pages.

For years, homoeopathy has been a system of profound healing, but one often limited by its subjectivity. The lack of standardized diagnosis, prognosis, and treatment planning tools has left practitioners with immense responsibility but without clear metrics for guidance. This realization led to the development of a framework—one that quantifies health, predicts curability, and guides treatment decisions with precision.

This book introduces a groundbreaking system of health scoring and curability assessment. Rooted in the principles of homoeopathy yet aligned with contemporary scientific methodologies, this framework seeks to bridge the gap between tradition and innovation. By offering a structured approach, it empowers practitioners to make confident decisions while fostering transparency and trust with patients.

The copyright recognition by the Government of India validates the significance of this work and serves as an inspiration to advance homoeopathy as a standardized, evidence-based practice. I hope this book becomes a cornerstone in modernizing homoeopathy and setting a benchmark for future innovations.

To the readers—whether you are a seasoned practitioner, a student, or an observer of homoeopathy—this book is an invitation to join a movement toward precision and standardization. Together, let us embrace this revolution and redefine the possibilities of healing.

Dr P Nidheesh

Author

Acknowledgements

This book is the result of a journey filled with inspiration, collaboration, and unwavering support from those who believe in the transformative power of homoeopathy. It is only fitting to express my deepest gratitude to those who have made this work possible.

First and foremost, I owe my deepest respect and appreciation to Dr. P. Radhakrishnan, my father, mentor, and a pioneer in the field of homoeopathy. His vision, profound dedication, and groundbreaking work have laid the foundation for this endeavor. His legacy in treating the most challenging cases with unparalleled success continues to inspire me every day.

To my colleagues and peers in homoeopathy, your discussions, feedback, and shared experiences have been invaluable. You have shaped the practical aspects of this work, ensuring its relevance and applicability to the challenges we face as practitioners.

To the patients who entrusted their care to me, I extend my heartfelt gratitude. Your trust and openness allowed me to refine and validate the concepts presented in this book. Your stories of resilience and recovery are a testament to the power of this system.

I am also deeply grateful to my family and friends for their unwavering support and encouragement throughout this journey. Your belief in me has been my anchor.

Finally, I acknowledge the Government of India for recognizing the originality and significance of this work through copyright protection. This achievement underscores the importance of advancing homoeopathy through innovation and scientific rigor.

To all who have walked this journey with me—directly or indirectly—thank you for being part of this revolution in homoeopathy.

With profound gratitude,
Dr P Nidheesh
Author

About The Author

Dr P. Nidheesh is a visionary homoeopath, philosopher, hypnotherapist, and international speaker whose pioneering work has redefined the landscape of homoeopathic medicine. As the son of the legendary Dr P. Radhakrishnan, Dr Nidheesh has seamlessly carried forward his father's legacy while carving out his own unique path in the world of homoeopathy.

Educational and Professional Background

Dr Nidheesh's academic journey reflects his deep commitment to mastering the art and science of homoeopathy. Armed with a comprehensive education in homoeopathic medicine and years of clinical experience, he has consistently pushed the boundaries of traditional practices to explore innovative methodologies.

Expertise Areas:

- Chronic and complex case management.
- Advanced homoeopathic therapeutics.
- Integrative approaches combining homoeopathy with modern scientific principles.
- Hypnotherapy for mind-body healing.
- A Researcher and Innovator

Dr Nidheesh is widely regarded as a trailblazer in homoeopathic research, with a particular focus on systematising and standardising treatment approaches. His development of The Hidden Protocol is a landmark achievement, bringing clarity and precision to a field often criticised for its subjectivity. This protocol, inspired by years of observing his father's unparalleled treatment methods, combines modern research with classical homoeopathic principles to empower practitioners worldwide.

A Thought Leader and International Speaker

Renowned for his engaging lectures and workshops, Dr Nidheesh has spoken at numerous international forums, inspiring homoeopaths to embrace evidence-based practices while preserving the essence of individualisation.

Philosophy:

Dr Nidheesh believes in the fusion of tradition and innovation, advocating for a balanced approach that respects the roots of homoeopathy while incorporating modern advancements.

Contributions to Homoeopathy

Dr Nidheesh's work goes beyond clinical practice; he is deeply invested in uplifting the homoeopathic community through education, mentorship, and philanthropy.

Key Contributions:

- Development of The Hidden Protocol, a standardised scoring system for treatment planning.
- Extensive research into disease curability, prognosis, and treatment methodologies.
- Advocacy for homoeopathy as a scientific, evidence-backed system of medicine.
- The Philosopher and Hypnotherapist

Beyond his role as a homoeopath, Dr Nidheesh is a trained hypnotherapist, blending mind-body healing techniques with homoeopathic principles. His philosophical insights add depth to his practice, ensuring his methods resonate with the whole person, not just their symptoms.

A Benevolent Visionary

Dr Nidheesh's ultimate goal is to empower homoeopaths worldwide, enabling them to treat patients with confidence, clarity, and compassion. He envisions a future where homoeopathy is globally recognised as a standardised and scientifically validated system of medicine. His work on The Hidden Protocol exemplifies this vision, offering practitioners a tool to deliver transformative care with precision and consistency.

Words from Dr Nidheesh

"Homoeopathy is not just medicine; it is the art of understanding the patient in their entirety. The Hidden Protocol is my humble effort to ensure that every homoeopath has the clarity and confidence to deliver this art with precision."

Dr P. Nidheesh continues to inspire and lead the homoeopathic community, proving that innovation rooted in tradition can elevate the field to unprecedented heights.

About Dr P Radhakrishnan

A Pillar of Homoeopathy

Dr P. Radhakrishnan is a name synonymous with excellence, compassion, and dedication in the field of homoeopathy. With over four decades of unparalleled service, he has touched the lives of countless patients, leaving an indelible mark on the medical community. As a retired Chief Medical Officer and the President of Inspire India NGO, Dr Radhakrishnan has devoted his life to the betterment of humanity through the healing art of homoeopathy.

A Storied Career

Beginning his journey in 1976, Dr Radhakrishnan's career spans decades of remarkable achievements and transformative contributions to homoeopathy. His practice has seen an extraordinary range of cases, from mild illnesses to the most severe and complex conditions, including cancer. His ability to apply homoeopathy to even the most challenging scenarios has earned him the admiration and respect of colleagues and patients alike.

Career Highlights:

- Successfully treated numerous cases of terminal illnesses, including cancer, showcasing the power of homoeopathy.
- Instrumental in integrating homoeopathy into mainstream healthcare through his government service.
- Renowned for his systematic, patient-centred approach that balances compassion with clinical precision.

A Leader in the Community

Dr Radhakrishnan's influence extends far beyond the consulting room. As the President of Inspire India NGO, he works tirelessly to promote healthcare accessibility and social welfare. His leadership in this role exemplifies his commitment to using his expertise to uplift communities and inspire others to do the same.

A Master Practitioner

Throughout his career, Dr Radhakrishnan has been recognised as a master practitioner of homoeopathy, blending scientific rigour with a deep understanding of the patient's individuality. His dedication to continuous learning and adaptation has enabled him to handle cases considered untreatable by conventional medicine.

Specialisations:

- Chronic and degenerative diseases.
- Palliative care with homoeopathy.
- Cases with multi-system involvement and advanced pathology.

An Inspiration to the Next Generation

Dr Radhakrishnan's influence is most profoundly seen in his role as a mentor and inspiration to the next generation of homoeopaths. His son, Dr P. Nidheesh, credits much of his success and vision to the wisdom and teachings of his father. Observing Dr Radhakrishnan's dedication and systematic approach inspired Dr Nidheesh to develop The Hidden Protocol, a tool designed to make his father's methods accessible to homoeopaths worldwide.

A Devotion to Homoeopathy

Dr Radhakrishnan's life's work is a testament to his unwavering belief in the transformative power of homoeopathy. He has not only dedicated himself to treating patients but has also tirelessly advocated for the global recognition of homoeopathy as a vital and effective system of medicine.

Legacy and Vision

Dr P. Radhakrishnan's legacy is one of excellence, dedication, and selflessness. His profound impact on homoeopathy will continue to inspire generations of practitioners, not only through his clinical success but also through the standardised treatment systems his methods have inspired.

Words from Dr P. Radhakrishnan

"Homoeopathy is more than just medicine; it is a way of life, a system that treats not just the body but the soul. My greatest joy has been to see lives transformed and suffering alleviated through this beautiful science."

Dr Radhakrishnan remains a beacon of hope and guidance, proving that with compassion, expertise, and a dedication to service, the boundaries of healing can be expanded infinitely.

Prologue

"Vision Statement

"To revolutionize and standardize homoeopathic treatment through the integration of 'The Hidden Protocol'—a structured scoring system that bridges classical principles and modern evidence-based practice."

Expanding the Vision

Homoeopathy, despite its widespread success, often faces criticism due to the lack of standardized treatment methodologies. Each practitioner interprets cases differently, leading to inconsistent outcomes. The Hidden Protocol seeks to resolve these disparities by offering a scientific, measurable, and reproducible approach to treatment.

Objectives of the Vision

- Enhance Precision in Diagnosis and Treatment

  - The protocol empowers practitioners to quantify patient health parameters systematically, minimizing subjective biases.

- Promote Consistency Across Practitioners

  - By implementing a scoring system, practitioners can align their methods with standardized metrics, ensuring uniform care.

- Integrate Modern Tools with Classical Wisdom

  - The system retains the essence of homoeopathic principles while incorporating modern analytical tools for a robust approach.

- Improve Patient Outcomes

  - A structured approach ensures accurate diagnosis, better treatment plans, and measurable progress tracking.

- Establish Credibility in Homoeopathy

  - Standardization through scoring can strengthen the scientific credibility of homoeopathy in the global medical community.

Why This Vision Matters

- Consistency: Homoeopathy often lacks uniformity in diagnosis and treatment, which can lead to scepticism. A scoring-based system offers consistency across practices.
- Transparency: By documenting and scoring case details, practitioners can communicate their decisions to patients and peers.
- Evidence-Based Practice: With measurable outcomes, The Hidden Protocol bridges the gap between traditional homoeopathy and modern clinical research.
- Empowerment: Practitioners gain confidence knowing their treatments are grounded in a reliable, repeatable framework.

How The Hidden Protocol Aligns with the Vision

As the documents outline, The Hidden Protocol offers a meticulous scoring system that evaluates various patient health parameters. By quantifying aspects such as intensity, duration, dreadfulness, and extent of disease, the protocol:

- Ensures holistic assessment.
- Guides practitioners toward appropriate remedies, dosages, and treatment plans.
- Differentiates between cases requiring palliation, symptomatic treatment, or similimum-based care.

"hidden" Protocol

HIDDEN stands for Health, Intensity, Duration, Dreadfulness, Extent, and Nature – six critical dimensions that define the essence of a patient's condition. These parameters, often overlooked or scattered across clinical observations, form a cohesive framework within The Hidden Protocol, offering a systematic approach to understanding the complexity of diseases.

Like a precious gem hidden within the layers of pathology, this protocol enables homoeopaths to unearth the true nature of a patient's illness. Each parameter is a key, unlocking a deeper understanding of the patient's health dynamics.

By decoding these elements, The Hidden Protocol empowers homoeopaths to move beyond superficial symptom management. It guides them to address the root cause of the disease with precision, crafting tailored treatment plans that align with the individual's unique presentation.

This tool is not just a protocol; it is a transformative methodology that bridges the gap between art and science in homoeopathy. It helps physicians connect the dots, revealing insights that are often obscured in clinical practice, and empowering them to confidently deliver cures that are lasting and profound.

Certificate Of Copyright Registration

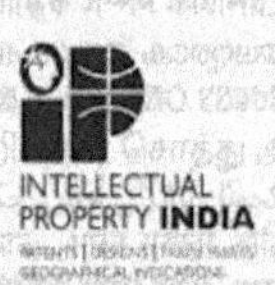

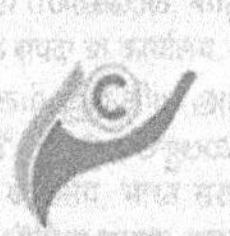

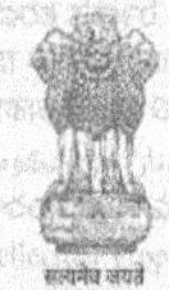

Extracts from the Register of Copyrights

प्रतिलिप्यधिकार कार्यालय, भारत सरकार | Copyright Office, Government Of India

fnukad/Dated:15/07/2024

1.	iathdj.k la[;k /Registration Number	:	**L-151085/2024**
2.	vkosnd dk uke] irk rFkk jk"V°h;rk Name, address and nationality of the applicant	:	DR P NIDHEESH , NEWLIFE HOMOEOPATHY CLINIC, VIYYUR , THRISSUR KERALA INDIA -680010 INDIAN OWNER
3.	—fr ds çfrfyf;f/kdkj esavkosnd ds fgr dh ç—fr Nature of the applicant's interest in the copyright of the work		
4.	—fr dk oxZ vkSj o.kZu Class and description of the work	:	LITERARY/ DRAMATIC WORK HIDDEN PROTOCOL A NEW TOOL TO IMPLEMENT STANDARDISATION IN HOMOEPATHIC PRACTICE
5.	—fr dk 'kh"kd Title of the work	:	HIDDEN PROTOCOL A NEW TOOL TO IMPLEMENT STANDARDISATION IN HOMOEPATHIC PRACTICE
6.	—fr dh Hkk"kk Language of the work	:	ENGLISH
7.	jpf;rk dk uke] irk vkSj jk"V°h;rk rFkk ;fn jpf;rk dh e`R;q gks xbZ gS] rks e`R;q dh frfFk Name, address and nationality of the author and if the author is deceased, date of his decease	:	DR P NIDHEESH , NEWLIFE HOMOEOPATHY CLINIC, VIYYUR , THRISSUR KERALA INDIA -680010 INDIAN
8.	—fr çdkf'kr gS ;k vçdkf'kr Whether the work is published or unpublished	:	UNPUBLISHED
9.	çFke çdk'ku dk o"kZ vkSj ns'k rFkk çdk'kd dk uke] irk vkSj jk"V°h;rk Year and country of first publication and name, address and nationality of the publisher	:	N.A.
10.	ckn ds çdk'kuksads o"kZ vkSj ns'k] ;fn dksbZ gksa] vkSj çdk'kdksads uke] irs vkSj jk"V°h;rk; Years and countries of subsequent publications, if any, and names, addresses and nationalities of the publishers	:	N.A.
11.	—fr esaçfrfyf;f/kdkj ifjgr fofHkUu vf/dkjksads Lokfe;ksads uke] irs vkSj jk"V°h;rk,vkSj leuqfs'ku vkSj vuqKfIr;ksads fooj.k ds IkFk çR;sd ds vf/kdkj dk foLrkj] ;fn dksbZ gksA Names, addresses and nationalities of the owners of various rights comprising the copyright in the work and the extent of rights held by each, together with particulars of assignments and licences, if any	:	DR P NIDHEESH , NEWLIFE HOMOEOPATHY CLINIC, VIYYUR , THRISSUR KERALA INDIA -680010 INDIAN
12.	vU; O;fa;ksads uke] irs vkSj jk"V°h;rk,a] ;fn dksbZ gksa] tks çfrfyf;f/kdkj okys vf/dkjksadks leuqfs'ku izir djus ;k vuqKfIr nsus ds fy, vf/k—r gksa Names, addresses and nationalities of other persons, if any, authorised to assign or licence of rights comprising the copyright	:	N.A.
13.	;fn —fr,d 'dykRed —fr gS] rks —fr ij vf/kdkj j[kus okys O;fa dk uke] irk vkSj jk"V°h;rk lfgr ewy —fr dk LFkkuA ¼,d okLrqf'kYi —fr ds ekeys esa—fr iwjh gksus dk o"kZ Hkh fn[kk;k tkuk pkfg,½ If the work is an 'Artistic work', the location of the original work, including name, address and nationality of the person in possession of the work. (In the case of an architectural work, the year of completion of the work should also be shown).	:	N.A.
14.	;fn —fr,d 'dykRed —fr gS tks fdlh Hkh eky ;k lsokvksads laca/k esa mi;ksx dh tkrh gS ;k mi;ksx fd, tkus esal{ke gS] rks vkosnu esa çfrfyf;f/kdkj vf/kfu;e] 1957 dh /kkjk 45 dh mi&/kkjk ¼i½ ds çko/kku ds vuqikji O;kikj fpà jftLV°kj ls çek.ku 'kkfey gksuk pkfg,A If the work is an 'Artistic work' which is used or capable of being used in relation to any goods or services, the application should include a certification from the Registrar of Trade Marks in terms of the provision to Sub-Section (i) of Section 45 of the Copyright Act, 1957.	:	N.A.
15.	;fn —fr,d 'dykRed —fr gS rks D;k ;g fMtkbu vf/kfu;e 2000 ds varxZr iath—r gS\ ;fn gka] rks fooj.k nsaA If the work is an 'Artistic work', whether it is registered under the Designs Act 2000, if yes give details.	:	N.A.
16.	;fn —fr,d 'dykRed —fr gS] tks fMtkbu vf/kfu;e 2000 ds rgr,d fMtkbu ds :i esaiath—r gksus esal{ke gS] rks D;k ;g vkS|ksfxd çfØ;k ds ek/;e ls fdlh olrq ij çxqä dh xbZ gS vkSj ;fn gka] rks bls fdruh ckj iqu#Rikfnr fd;k x;k gS\ If the work is an 'Artistic work', capable of being registered as a design under the Designs Act 2000.whether it has been applied to an article though an industrial process and ,if yes ,the number of times it is reproduced.	:	N.A.
17.	fVIi.kh] ;fn dksbZ gks/Remarks, if any	:	

Mk;jh la[;k/Diary Number: 13559/2024-CO/L

vkosnu dh frfFk/Date of Application: 29/04/2024

çkfIr dh frfFk/Date of Receipt: 29/04/2024

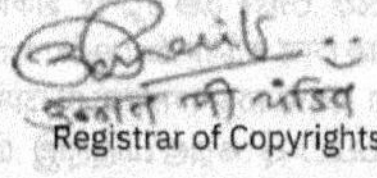

Registrar of Copyrights

COPYRIGHT CERTIFICATE

ONE

THE NEED FOR A SCORING SYSTEM IN HOMOEOPATHY

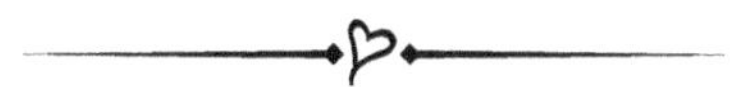

Introduction

Homoeopathy, since its inception, has relied predominantly on qualitative assessments of patient symptoms, remedy selection, and case prognosis. While this method fosters deep individualisation, it remains largely subjective and dependent on practitioner experience. As the global movement toward evidence-based medicine accelerates, the lack of quantifiable tools in homoeopathy has emerged as a critical gap. A structured scoring system offers a transformative solution by bridging the art of individualisation with the precision of objective measurement.

Limitations of Traditional Homoeopathic Case Evaluation

- Despite its unparalleled depth, classical homoeopathy presents several practical challenges:
- Subjectivity: Interpretation of symptoms, remedy selection, and prognosis often varies between practitioners.
- Lack of reproducibility: Different doctors may arrive at different conclusions for the same case, even when applying the same philosophical principles.
- Difficulty in Monitoring Progress: Evaluating whether a case is improving or worsening is often described narratively rather than through quantifiable parameters.
- Challenges in Research and Standardisation: Without numerical data, it becomes difficult to conduct large-scale research, compare cases, or establish treatment protocols.
- These challenges highlight the urgent need for a reproducible, semi-quantitative model that retains individualisation while introducing objectivity.

The Role of a Scoring System

- A scoring system in homoeopathy is designed to serve multiple purposes:
- Quantify Patient State: By assigning scores to symptom intensity, pathology severity, miasmatic dominance, vitality, and other clinical parameters, the patient's condition can be mapped systematically.
- Standardise Case-taking and Analysis: Scoring ensures that important aspects are not overlooked and are evaluated systematically across different cases and practitioners.
- Facilitate Remedy Selection: Remedies could be matched based not only on symptom similarity but also by fitting the biological, psychological, and pathological profile emerging from scores.
- Track Case Progress Objectively: By comparing scores over time, practitioners can objectively measure improvement, standstill, or deterioration.
- Aid Research: Statistical analyses become feasible when cases are presented with numerical scoring, opening doors for evidence-based validation of homoeopathic approaches.
- Enhance Training: Young homoeopaths can be guided systematically in evaluating cases, thus reducing early errors due to inexperience.

- Support Communication: Scoring offers a common language for interdisciplinary discussions, including communication with conventional medical practitioners.

Principles of Designing a Homoeopathic Scoring System
For a scoring system to be effective and true to the homoeopathic spirit, it must:

- Respect Individualisation: Scoring should capture the uniqueness of each patient rather than forcing rigid classification.
- Be Flexible Yet Standardised: It should have a defined framework but allow adjustments based on the depth of each case.
- Incorporate Multi-dimensionality: Physical, emotional, mental, pathological, and miasmatic aspects should be separately scored to create a holistic view.
- Allow Dynamic Monitoring: The system must accommodate the evolving nature of disease and health during treatment.
- Be Simple Yet Scientifically Robust: Practitioners should be able to apply it practically without feeling burdened, while also ensuring scientific credibility.

TWO

OVERVIEW OF "THE HIDDEN PROTOCOL"

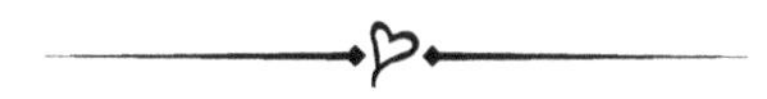

What is "The Hidden Protocol"?

The Hidden Protocol is an innovative, structured scoring system developed to standardize homoeopathic treatment while preserving the essence of classical individualisation. Integrating the foundational principles of traditional homoeopathy with a modern, evidence-based framework, it provides a systematic method for evaluating, scoring, and treating patients holistically.

By deconstructing complex patient presentations into quantifiable components, The Hidden Protocol enhances consistency, objectivity, and precision in clinical practice — thus representing a paradigm shift in the field of homoeopathy.

Key Components of "The Hidden Protocol"

The system is organised into carefully defined domains that collectively provide a comprehensive view of the patient:

1. Patient Information

- The initial framework gathers fundamental demographic and physiological data, including age, sex, occupation, and detailed medical history. This ensures an individualized assessment that recognises constitutional influences and predisposing factors.

2. General Parameters

- Routine physiological functions—such as appetite, thirst, stool, urine, perspiration, sleep, and menstrual health—are systematically evaluated. These general symptoms serve as windows into the organism's homeostatic balance and adaptive capacity.

3. Mental Generals

The cognitive and intellectual dimensions of the patient are assessed, encompassing:

- Awareness of capabilities,
- Resilience to stress,
- Performance efficiency.

This evaluation helps determine the degree of psychological integration or fragmentation, which influences both disease susceptibility and remedy response.

4. Emotional Attributes

- The patient's emotional terrain is meticulously analysed, focusing on:
- Stability versus volatility of emotions,
- Predominance of negative emotional states,
- Influence of emotional disturbances on physical pathology.

This domain captures the vital dynamism of the patient, offering critical clues for remedy individualisation.

5. Disease Parameters

The pathology is rigorously profiled based on:

- Intensity of symptoms,
- Chronicity and duration,
- Dreadfulness (functional and pathological severity),
- Extent of systemic involvement,
- Nature of progression (self-limiting, degenerative, destructive).

This enables precise disease staging and informs prognosis and treatment planning.

How the Scoring System Works

Each parameter within the protocol is assigned a numeric score according to the severity, peculiarity, or deviation it presents.

The scores across all domains are then aggregated to generate a composite health profile. This system enables practitioners to:

- Prioritise key aspects influencing case management,
- Objectively distinguish between self-limiting and intervention-requiring conditions,
- Identify when palliation or surgical referral becomes necessary,
- Strategically align remedy selection, potency, and repetition to the case dynamics.
- The scoring structure thus creates a scientifically valid pathway between symptom observation and therapeutic action.

In essence, The Hidden Protocol elevates homoeopathic practice to a new standard — one that honours Hahnemannian wisdom while embracing the demands of contemporary medical science.

The Hidden Protocol represents a landmark advancement in the evolution of homoeopathy.

By synergising classical principles with a rigorously defined, scientific methodology, it brings unprecedented clarity, reproducibility, and effectiveness to case management.

In doing so, it lays the foundation for a globally standardised, research-compatible model of homoeopathic care — ensuring that homoeopathy not only retains its timeless relevance but also achieves its rightful place within the modern healthcare ecosystem.

THREE

FOUNDATIONS OF THE HIDDEN PROTOCOL

Reimagining Holistic Healing

At its core, The Hidden Protocol is a response to the need for a systematic, yet individualized, approach to homoeopathic treatment. Traditional homoeopathy, while effective, often relies heavily on the subjective interpretation of symptoms. This can lead to inconsistencies and variable outcomes. The Hidden Protocol provides a framework to eliminate these challenges, rooted in three core principles:

Classical Homoeopathy

Anchored in the principles of symptom similarity and individualization, homoeopathy has always sought to treat the person rather than the disease.

The Hidden Protocol preserves this essence by ensuring that the scoring system reflects the unique aspects of a patient's condition.

Modern Evidence-Based Medicine

Contemporary healthcare demands quantifiable and reproducible methods.

This protocol introduces measurable parameters into the diagnostic and treatment process, bridging the gap between traditional practices and modern expectations.

Systematic Case Evaluation

By transforming qualitative observations into quantifiable data, the protocol ensures that practitioners can evaluate and compare cases with precision.

This systematic approach fosters consistency, making outcomes predictable and scientifically valid.

Core Foundations

Holistic Perspective

The protocol treats health as a dynamic balance influenced by:

- Physical symptoms.
- Mental and emotional states.
- Environmental factors.

This integrative approach ensures that no aspect of the patient's well-being is overlooked.

Patient-Centred Philosophy

- Each individual's journey to health is unique. The protocol acknowledges this by adapting its methodology to the patient's specific needs.
- It encourages active patient involvement, fostering trust and collaboration in the healing process.

Data-Driven Insights

- Quantifiable metrics offer clarity, enabling practitioners to make informed decisions.
- The protocol allows practitioners to track progress, refine treatment plans, and showcase measurable improvements.

Scalability and Flexibility

- Whether addressing a simple acute case or a complex chronic condition, the protocol adapts to varying levels of complexity.
- Its design accommodates diverse medical scenarios, ensuring broad applicability.

Bridging Traditional and Modern Practices

Homoeopathy has long been regarded as an art—relying on the practitioner's intuition and experience. However, modern medicine emphasizes the importance of reproducibility and objectivity. The Hidden Protocol successfully integrates these paradigms:

- Retaining the individualized care of traditional homoeopathy.
- Incorporating standardized metrics to meet modern scientific standards.
- Supporting clinical research with measurable outcomes.
- Empowering Practitioners

By adopting The Hidden Protocol, practitioners gain:

- Confidence in their diagnoses and treatment plans.
- Credibility through adherence to a structured, validated system.
- Efficiency in evaluating and managing cases systematically.
- Empathy by maintaining a focus on the patient's holistic well-being.

> "*The Hidden Protocol stands on the firm foundations of homoeopathic philosophy, enriched with modern scientific rigor. It is a tool designed to elevate the practice of homoeopathy, ensuring that practitioners can deliver consistent, effective, and patient-centered care.*"

FOUR

PHILOSOPHY BEHIND THE PROTOCOL

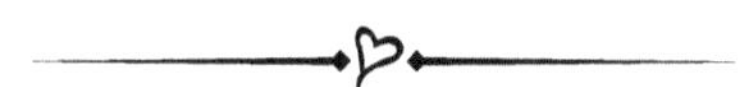

The Core Philosophy

The Hidden Protocol is underpinned by a unifying principle: the advancement of homoeopathy as a precise, evidence-based, and patient-centred system of medicine. By integrating the art of homoeopathy with scientific methodologies, the protocol bridges the longstanding divide between traditional wisdom and modern medical practices.

At its heart, this philosophy espouses:

- *Holism*

  - Recognising the intricate interplay between physical, mental, and emotional dimensions of health, the protocol ensures that all facets of the patient are taken into account.

- *Standardisation with Flexibility*

  - While embracing the need for reproducibility in clinical settings, the protocol maintains the flexibility required to honour the uniqueness of each patient.

- *Healing Beyond Symptom Suppression*

  - The emphasis is placed on stimulating the body's inherent healing mechanisms, rather than merely masking symptoms, aligning with the foundational principles of homoeopathy.

- *Empowerment through Clarity*

  - By offering practitioners a structured framework, the protocol enhances diagnostic precision, therapeutic confidence, and transparency in patient communication.

Key Tenets of the Protocol's Philosophy

- *Patient-Centric Individualisation*

  - Each patient's health journey is unique, shaped by their genetics, environment, lifestyle, and mental state.
  - The protocol provides a scoring mechanism that accommodates these variables, ensuring truly personalised care.

- *Dynamic Nature of Disease*

  - The progression of disease is fluid, and influenced by internal and external factors.
  - The protocol reflects this by incorporating dynamic parameters such as intensity, duration, and emotional impact into its scoring system.

- *Balancing Tradition and Evidence*

  - Homoeopathy has long been regarded as an art; however, modern medicine demands evidence-based practices.
  - The protocol's scoring model provides measurable outcomes, thus bridging this critical gap.

- *Transparency and Accountability*

  - The ability to quantify health parameters enhances the transparency of therapeutic decisions, fostering trust between practitioner and patient.

Philosophical Alignment with Homoeopathy
The Hidden Protocol is firmly rooted in the classical principles of homoeopathy:

- Similia Similibus Curentur (Like Cures Like)

  - Remedies are selected based on a holistic understanding of the patient, ensuring alignment with this cornerstone of homoeopathic philosophy.

- Vital Force Restoration

  - By evaluating the mental, emotional, and physical dimensions of health, the protocol works to restore equilibrium in the vital force—a key concept in homoeopathy.

- Individualisation with Precision

  - The scoring system ensures that no two patients are treated alike, honouring the homoeopathic emphasis on individualised care while providing a consistent framework.

Guiding Principles

- From Symptom Observation to Systemic Analysis

  - The protocol moves beyond symptomatic relief, facilitating a deeper understanding of the underlying systemic imbalances.

- From Complexity to Clarity

  - The inherent complexity of chronic and multi-layered cases is distilled into actionable insights through structured scoring.

- From Cure to Comprehensive Care

- While aiming for curative outcomes, the protocol equally prioritises palliative and preventative strategies where curative treatment is unattainable.

"The Hidden Protocol embodies a philosophy of transformation within homoeopathy. It introduces a scientifically robust yet profoundly humanistic approach to patient care, underscoring the practitioner's role as both a healer and a clinical scientist. By combining timeless principles with contemporary tools, the protocol paves the way for a future where homoeopathy is both respected and standardised globally."

FIVE

THE EVOLUTION OF THE HIDDEN PROTOCOL

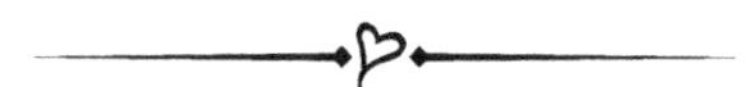

Origins of the Protocol

The Hidden Protocol was conceived as a response to longstanding challenges in homoeopathy: the need for greater standardisation, measurable outcomes, and enhanced credibility within the broader medical community. Its development is a testament to the integration of classical homoeopathic principles with the demands of modern clinical practice.

Recognition of Challenges

- Inconsistent treatment outcomes due to subjective interpretation of symptoms.
- Limited acceptance of homoeopathy in evidence-based medical frameworks.
- Difficulties in managing complex cases with overlapping symptoms or chronic conditions.

Visionary Beginnings

Aimed at addressing these gaps, the protocol was initially designed to organise the complexity of homoeopathic case-taking into a structured, replicable framework.

Milestones in Development

- *Conceptualisation*

  - The foundational principles of the protocol were derived from the practice of classical homoeopathy, with a focus on individualisation, dynamic analysis, and holistic treatment.
  - Early iterations involved mapping traditional homoeopathic methodologies to measurable parameters.

- *Collaboration and Refinement*

  - The protocol was refined through collaboration with leading homoeopaths and researchers, ensuring its alignment with clinical realities and academic rigour.
  - Feedback from practitioners highlighted the need for simplicity and adaptability in the scoring mechanism.

- *Validation Through Practice*

  - The protocol was rigorously tested across a variety of cases, ranging from acute conditions to chronic, multi-layered disorders.
  - Comparative studies demonstrated improved consistency in treatment outcomes when using the protocol.

- *Integration of Modern Tools*

  - Advances in data analytics, psychology, and medical research were incorporated into the protocol, ensuring its relevance in contemporary practice.
  - Features such as curability scoring, disease intensity levels, and treatment pathways were introduced to enhance its utility.

Key Phases of Evolution

- *Early Framework (Phase 1)*

  - Focused on simplifying case-taking by organising patient data into structured categories.
  - Emphasised the importance of quantifying general and mental symptoms.

- *Advanced Scoring Models (Phase 2)*

  - Introduced weighted scoring for parameters such as emotional impact, intensity, and duration of symptoms.
  - Established correlations between scores and treatment outcomes, enhancing predictive accuracy.

- *Integration with Clinical Research (Phase 3)*

  - Applied in real-world clinical settings to validate efficacy and adaptability.
  - Data collected from these studies reinforced the protocol's utility in achieving reproducible results.

- *Final Model (Phase 4)*

  - A comprehensive scoring system encompassing physical, mental, emotional, and disease-specific parameters.
  - Designed for seamless integration into both solo practices and institutional settings.

A Revolutionary Impact

- *Empowering Practitioners*

  - The Hidden Protocol equips homoeopaths with a tool that enhances their diagnostic precision and therapeutic confidence, fostering professional growth.

- *Improving Patient Outcomes*

  - By prioritising individualisation within a standardised framework, the protocol ensures that patients receive care tailored to their unique needs.

- *Advancing Homoeopathy*

  - Through its evidence-based approach, the protocol strengthens homoeopathy's position within integrative medicine, enabling dialogue with other medical disciplines.

"The evolution of The Hidden Protocol reflects a journey of innovation and collaboration. It has transformed from a conceptual framework into a robust, validated system that addresses the challenges of modern homoeopathy

while staying true to its philosophical roots. The next section will delve into the scientific and clinical foundations that underpin this revolutionary approach."

SIX

SCIENTIFIC AND CLINICAL FOUNDATIONS

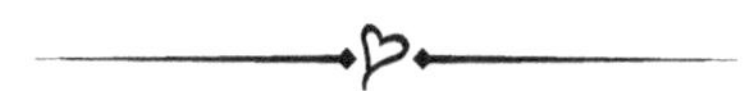

"The Hidden Protocol is firmly grounded in a dual foundation: the philosophical tenets of classical homoeopathy and the rigorous demands of modern scientific methodology. This section outlines the scientific principles, clinical evidence, and data-driven insights that validate and enhance the protocol's effectiveness."

1. Evidence-Based Roots

Homoeopathy has often faced criticism for its lack of standardisation and quantifiable outcomes. The Hidden Protocol addresses these critiques by incorporating:

Quantifiable Parameters

- Parameters such as symptom intensity, disease duration, and emotional impact are scored systematically.
- This approach transforms subjective observations into measurable data, enabling consistency and reproducibility.

Validation Through Clinical Experience

- Clinical trials and retrospective studies have demonstrated the protocol's utility in improving diagnostic accuracy and treatment outcomes.
- Data from case studies confirm the predictive value of its scoring system, particularly in identifying curable and palliative cases.

2. Clinical Application and Outcomes

The Hidden Protocol has been tested in a variety of clinical scenarios, including:

- Acute Cases

  - For short-term, self-limiting conditions, the protocol simplifies the identification of appropriate remedies by scoring general and mental symptoms.
  - Example: A patient with acute respiratory distress scored high on intensity and emotional stress, leading to precise remedy selection. Improvement was observed within 12 hours.

- Chronic and Complex Cases

  - Chronic conditions often involve multi-system involvement and overlapping symptoms. The protocol's scoring mechanism aids in breaking down these complexities.

- Example: A patient with rheumatoid arthritis and depression was scored across physical and emotional parameters, leading to a combined approach of constitutional remedies and lifestyle modifications.

- Paediatric Cases

  - Children often present with subtle symptoms that require careful interpretation. The protocol's objective scoring system ensures accurate assessments.
  - Example: A paediatric case of recurrent tonsillitis scored high on susceptibility and emotional distress, guiding effective treatment.

3. Alignment with Modern Medicine

The protocol establishes a bridge between homoeopathy and contemporary healthcare by:

- Integrating Pathology

  - By incorporating parameters such as disease intensity and pathology levels, the protocol aligns with conventional medical diagnostics while maintaining homoeopathic principles.

- Curability and Prognosis

  - The scoring system offers insights into the curability of cases, providing a scientific basis for prognosis and patient counselling.
  - Example: Patients with high curability scores often show faster recovery and fewer relapses.

- Reproducibility

  - The structured framework ensures that cases can be evaluated and treated with consistency across practitioners and institutions.

4. Scientific Underpinnings

- The Hidden Protocol draws on multiple scientific disciplines, including:

  - Psychoneuroimmunology
  - By recognising the interplay between emotional health and immunity, the protocol emphasises the importance of mental and emotional parameters in treatment.

- Systems Biology

  - The holistic approach of the protocol aligns with systems biology, which views the body as an interconnected network rather than an isolated organ system.

- Data Science

  - The protocol's scoring system is designed to generate data that can be analysed to identify patterns, predict outcomes, and refine treatment methodologies.

5. Bridging Research and Practice

- ***For Practitioners***

  - Practitioners gain a tool that enhances clinical decision-making through clear metrics and structured evaluation.

- ***For Patients***

  - Patients benefit from transparent, predictable, and evidence-based treatment plans that foster trust and collaboration.

- ***For Academia and Research***

  - The protocol provides a framework for conducting reproducible studies, paving the way for greater acceptance of homoeopathy in integrative medicine.

  "The scientific and clinical foundations of The Hidden Protocol exemplify its transformative potential. By combining evidence-based methodologies with homoeopathy's holistic philosophy, the protocol sets a new standard for practice and research. The subsequent sections will delve into the detailed mechanics of the scoring system and its application in real-world scenarios."

SEVEN
OBJECTIVES OF THE SCORING SYSTEM

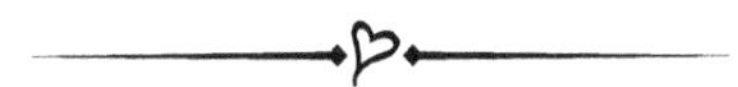

"The scoring system within The Hidden Protocol represents a paradigm shift in homoeopathic practice, bridging the art of individualisation with the precision of standardisation. This section elucidates the primary objectives of this system, which serves as the cornerstone of modernised homoeopathic case-taking and management."

1. Standardisation of Case Evaluation

- Consistency Across Practitioners:

  - The scoring system provides a uniform framework, ensuring that homoeopaths evaluate cases using consistent criteria.
  - Example: A case of chronic asthma scored by two practitioners will yield comparable assessments, enabling shared understanding and collaboration.

- Reproducibility:

  - The structured approach transforms subjective impressions into objective metrics, facilitating reproducible results in clinical and research settings.

2. Quantification of Subjective Observations

- From Qualitative to Quantitative:

  - Patient-reported symptoms and practitioner-observed signs, which are inherently subjective, are systematically quantified using defined scales.
  - Example: Anxiety is not simply noted but scored based on severity and impact, providing measurable data for treatment planning.

- Enhanced Precision:

  - Quantification minimises bias, enabling homoeopaths to focus on the most critical aspects of a case.

3. Facilitation of Clinical Decision-Making

- Guidance on Remedy Selection:

  - The scores highlight the dominant themes in a case, such as emotional distress or severe pathology, guiding remedy selection and potency decisions.
  - Example: A high score in emotional attributes may direct attention to remedies addressing grief, fear, or frustration.

- Prognostic Insights:

  - The scoring system offers clarity on the curability of a case, aiding in setting realistic expectations for patients.

- Treatment Pathway Definition:

  - Each case level, determined by the aggregated score, corresponds to specific treatment strategies, ranging from simple symptom similarity to complex miasmatic and pathological considerations.

4. Transparency and Accountability

- Objective Reporting:

  - The scoring system enables practitioners to present their findings transparently to patients and peers, building trust and accountability.
  - Example: Sharing a patient's curability percentage with them fosters confidence in the treatment plan.

- Peer Validation:

  - The structured approach allows for easier review and validation of cases by other homoeopaths, enhancing collaborative learning and practice.

5. Prediction of Outcomes

- Curability Assessment:

  - By correlating scores with historical data and clinical evidence, the protocol predicts the likelihood of recovery or palliation.
  - Example: A case with a high disease score but moderate emotional scores may indicate a longer treatment course but a promising outcome.

- Treatment Adjustments:

  - Periodic rescoring during follow-ups enables practitioners to track progress objectively and adjust treatment plans as necessary.

6. Enabling Data-Driven Homoeopathy

- Research Opportunities:

- ◦ Aggregated scores from multiple cases provide a rich database for analysing treatment efficacy, remedy selection patterns, and disease trends.

- Integrating Technology:

  - ◦ The protocol's structured design lends itself to integration with digital tools, such as electronic health records and decision-support systems.

"The scoring system is not merely a tool but a transformative framework that elevates the practice of homoeopathy to new levels of precision and scientific rigour. By standardising evaluations, quantifying observations, and facilitating clear decision-making, it empower practitioners to deliver more effective and transparent care."

DECODING THE HIDDEN PROTOCOL

EIGHT

CORE COMPONENTS OF THE SCORING SYSTEM

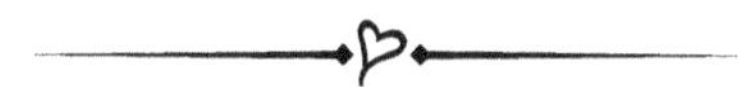

"The scoring system of The Hidden Protocol is a meticulously designed framework that captures the complexity of homoeopathic case evaluation. It is built upon four primary domains, each encompassing a range of parameters critical to understanding and managing a patient's condition."

1. General Parameters

These parameters assess the physiological balance and functionality of the patient's bodily systems. They include:

- Appetite

    - Evaluates regularity and abnormalities in hunger patterns.
    - Scoring: 0 (Normal) to 0.5 (Reduced or excessive).

- Thirst

    - Monitors hydration patterns, focusing on excessive or reduced intake.
    - Scoring: 0 (Normal) to 0.5 (Abnormal).

- Stool and Urine

    - Analyses elimination processes for irregularities such as constipation, diarrhoea, or discolouration.
    - Scoring: 0 (Normal) to 0.5 (Abnormal).

- Sweat

    - Assesses the appropriateness of sweating patterns, including minimal or excessive perspiration.
    - Scoring: 0 (Normal) to 0.5 (Abnormal).

- Sleep

    - Focuses on consistency and quality of rest, including disturbances like insomnia or hypersomnia.
    - Scoring: 0 (Normal) to 0.5 (Abnormal).

2. Mental and Emotional Attributes

This domain evaluates the patient's psychological state and its impact on health. It includes:

- Awareness of Abilities

  - Measures self-perception and understanding of personal capabilities.
  - Scoring: 0 (Well Aware) to 2 (Not Aware).

- Stress-Coping Ability

  - Assesses how well the patient manages stressors.
  - Scoring: 0 (Well Coped) to 2 (Cannot Cope).

- Productivity and Fruitfulness

  - Evaluates the patient's functional output and life satisfaction.
  - Scoring: 0 (Good) to 2 (Unproductive).

- Emotional Scale

  - Captures the intensity of emotional states, ranging from positivity to severe negativity (e.g., joy to despair).
  - Scoring: 0 (Positive Emotions) to 2 (Severe Negative Emotions).

- Mental Attributes Contributing to Illness

  - Identifies whether mental factors exacerbate physical conditions.
  - Scoring: 0 (No Contribution) to 2 (Significant Contribution).

3. Disease-Specific Parameters
These parameters provide insights into the condition's severity and progression:

- Intensity

  - Measures the severity of the presenting symptoms.
  - Scoring: 1 (Mild) to 6 (Life-threatening).

- Duration

  - Tracks the length of time the condition has persisted.
  - Scoring: 1 (<10 days) to 6 (>3 years).

- Dreadfulness of Disease

  - Categorises the disease based on its pathology and potential impact.
  - Scoring: 1 (Reversible without medication) to 6 (Irreversible requiring palliation).

- Extent of Disease

  - Evaluates the breadth of involvement, from a single organ to multi-system diseases.

- Scoring: 1 (Superficial Organ) to 6 (Metastasis or Multi-system).

- Nature of Disease

  - Differentiates between self-limiting and chronic conditions requiring intervention.
  - Scoring: 1 (Self-limiting) to 6 (Permanent deformity or palliation required).

4. Historical and Lifestyle Factors
Understanding the patient's background is crucial for accurate treatment planning. This domain includes:

- Past History

  - Assesses previous illnesses and their impact on the current condition.
  - Scoring: 0 (No History) to 2 (Very Strong History).

- Family History

  - Evaluates hereditary predispositions to illnesses.
  - Scoring: 0 (No History) to 2 (Very Strong History).

- Treatment History

  - Analyses the effectiveness and continuation of previous treatments.
  - Scoring: 0 (No History) to 2 (Very Strong History).

- Personal Habits and Stress

  - Considers lifestyle factors such as diet, exercise, and stress levels.
  - Scoring: 0 (No Impact) to 2 (Significant Impact).

"The four domains of the scoring system provide a comprehensive view of the patient, blending subjective insights with objective data. Each domain contributes to a holistic understanding, ensuring that no aspect of the patient's condition is overlooked. This systematic approach enables practitioners to deliver precise and personalised care."

NINE

APPETITE

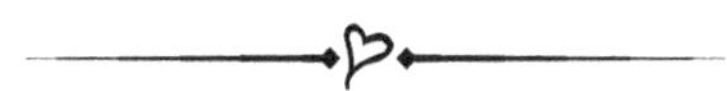

Appetite

Appetite refers to the psychological desire to eat, which is influenced by a complex interplay of physiological, psychological, and environmental factors. Unlike hunger, which is a physiological need for food, appetite is more subjective and can be stimulated by sensory cues or emotions.

Normal Appetite

1. **Regulation:** Normal appetite reflects the body's ability to signal hunger and satiety through hormonal and neural pathways. Key hormones include ghrelin (stimulating appetite) and leptin (indicating satiety).
2. **Stimuli:** Appetite is triggered by sensory cues like the sight, smell, or thought of food, alongside physical activity and time since the last meal.
3. **Consistency:** A normal appetite fluctuates with energy needs but aligns with maintaining a stable body weight and nutritional balance.

Abnormal Appetite

1. **Increased Appetite (Hyperphagia):**

   - **Definition:** Excessive hunger or eating beyond the body's energy requirements.

   - **Causes:** Conditions such as hyperthyroidism, diabetes mellitus, or psychological factors like binge eating disorder.
   - **Impact:** Can lead to obesity and associated metabolic disorders.

1. Decreased Appetite (Hypophagia or Anorexia):

   - **Definition:** Reduced desire to eat or inability to maintain adequate energy intake.

   - **Causes:** Chronic illnesses (e.g., cancer, gastrointestinal disorders), depression, or side effects of medications.
   - **Impact:** May result in malnutrition, weight loss, and impaired immunity.

3. Fluctuating Appetite:

- **Definition:** Irregular patterns of appetite influenced by stress, hormonal imbalances, or lifestyle factors.

- **Causes:** Premenstrual syndrome, pregnancy, or eating disorders like bulimia nervosa.

TEN
THIRST

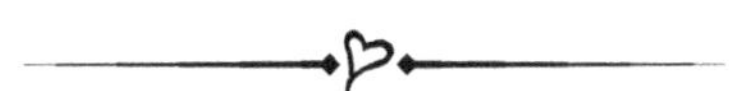

Thirst

Thirst is a natural physiological mechanism driven by the body's need to maintain fluid balance and regulate homeostasis. It serves as a critical signal for fluid intake, ensuring proper hydration for cellular and systemic functions.

Normal Thirst

1. **Regulation:** Thirst is primarily controlled by the hypothalamus in response to changes in plasma osmolality or blood volume. An increase in osmolality or a decrease in blood volume triggers the sensation of thirst.
2. **Stimuli:** Normal thirst is typically stimulated by dehydration, increased physical activity, high dietary salt intake, or hot environmental conditions.
3. **Pattern:** A normal response to thirst involves drinking water or other fluids sufficient to restore hydration. Once fluid balance is achieved, thirst subsides.

Abnormal Thirst

1. **Excessive Thirst (Polydipsia):**

   - **Definition:** Excessive and persistent urge to drink fluids, often beyond the body's needs.
   - **Causes:** Common causes include diabetes mellitus (due to increased glucose-induced osmotic diuresis), diabetes insipidus (due to lack of antidiuretic hormone), or psychological conditions such as psychogenic polydipsia.
   - **Impact:** Can lead to overhydration, electrolyte imbalances, and associated complications.

2. Decreased Thirst (Adipsia):

   - **Definition:** Reduced or absent sensation of thirst, even in the presence of dehydration.

   - **Causes:** Often associated with hypothalamic dysfunction, brain injuries, or neurological conditions.
   - **Impact:** Can result in dehydration, hypotension, and impaired thermoregulation.

1. Abnormal Thirst Patterns:

- ◦ **Definition:** Thirst patterns that do not correlate with physiological needs, such as craving fluids without dehydration or not drinking enough despite high fluid loss
- ◦ **Causes:** Could be due to medications (e.g., diuretics), excessive salt intake, or disorders affecting thirst regulation

ELEVEN

BLADDER HABITS

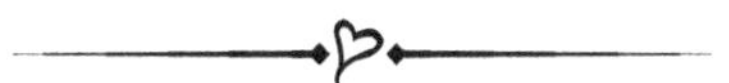

Bladder habits include the frequency, volume, and control of urination. Recognising what constitutes normal and abnormal patterns is essential for identifying potential health concerns.

Normal Bladder Habits

1. **Frequency:** Adults typically urinate 5–7 times during the day and no more than once at night. This can vary based on fluid intake, age, and other factors .
2. **Volume:** A healthy bladder can hold about 300–500 mL of urine and empties approximately 200–300 mL per void.
3. **Control:** Normal bladder control means the ability to delay urination until a convenient time without discomfort or leakage.

Abnormal Bladder Habits

1. **Increased Frequency (Polyuria):** Urinating more than 8 times in 24 hours may indicate overactive bladder, diabetes, or urinary tract infections.
2. **Nocturia:** Waking more than once at night to urinate can suggest bladder overactivity or heart or kidney conditions.
3. **Urgency:** A sudden, strong urge to urinate that is difficult to postpone is abnormal and may indicate overactive bladder or irritation.
4. **Incontinence:** Any involuntary leakage of urine is abnormal and could be due to stress or urge incontinence.
5. **Retention:** Difficulty initiating urination or the sensation of incomplete bladder emptying suggests underactive bladder or retention issues.

TWELVE
BOWEL HABITS

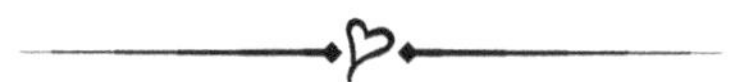

Bowel habits refer to the frequency, consistency, and ease of stool passage, which are critical indicators of gastrointestinal health. Variations in bowel habits may be normal, but persistent abnormalities often suggest underlying health issues.

Normal Bowel Habits

1. **Frequency:**

   ◦ 1 to 3 times per day or 3 times per week, depending on individual variation.

1. Consistency (Bristol Stool Chart Types 3–4):

   ◦ Smooth, soft, and easy-to-pass stools.

3. Other Characteristics:

   ◦ Minimal effort required for defecation.

   ◦ No associated pain, bloating, or discomfort.

   ◦ Stools are free of blood or mucus.

Abnormal Bowel Habits

1. **Frequency:**

   ◦ **Infrequent (Constipation):** Fewer than 3 bowel movements per week.

   ◦ **Frequent (Diarrhoea):** More than 3 loose or watery stools per day.

2. Consistency (Bristol Stool Chart Types 1–2 or 5–7):

   ◦ **Hard or Lumpy (Constipation):** Difficulty passing stools.

   ◦ **Watery or Mushy (Diarrhoea):** Rapid stool passage, often with urgency .

3. Other Abnormalities:

   ◦ Presence of blood, mucus, or undigested food in stools.

   ◦ Pain, bloating, or discomfort during defecation.

   ◦ Incomplete evacuation or excessive straining.
   ◦ Changes in colour, such as black (melena) or pale stools, indicating potential pathology

Normal vs Abnormal Stool Characteristics

Frequency:

- Normal: 1–3 times per day to 3 times per week
- Abnormal: Less than 3 times per week (constipation) or more than 3 times per day (diarrhoea)

Consistency:

- Normal: Smooth, soft (Bristol Stool Types 3–4)
- Abnormal: Hard, lumpy (Types 1–2) or watery (Types 5–7)

Effort:

- Normal: Minimal effort required
- Abnormal: Presence of straining or urgency

Associated Symptoms:

- Normal: None
- Abnormal: Pain, bloating, blood, or mucus in stools

THIRTEEN

PERSPIRATION

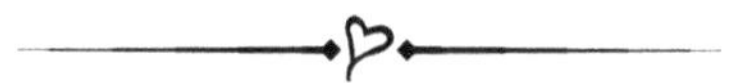

Perspiration, also known as sweating, is the body's natural mechanism to regulate temperature and maintain homeostasis. It involves the secretion of sweat from sweat glands, primarily in response to heat, physical activity, or stress.

Normal Perspiration

1. **Function:** Sweating helps regulate body temperature by evaporative cooling and eliminates small amounts of waste products, including salt and urea (1).
2. **Triggering Factors:** Normal perspiration is typically stimulated by:

   - **Environmental heat:** Increased temperatures activate thermoregulatory mechanisms.

   - **Physical activity:** Exercise-induced sweating helps cool the body during exertion.

   - **Emotional stress:** Emotional or nervous stimuli can activate apocrine sweat glands (2).

2. **Volume:** The average person secretes 500–700 mL of sweat daily under normal conditions. This amount can increase to several litres during intense physical activity or heat exposure (3).

Abnormal Perspiration

Excessive Sweating (Hyperhidrosis):

- **Definition:** Sweating beyond what is required for thermoregulation.

- Types:

  - **Primary (Focal) Hyperhidrosis:** Localised to areas such as palms, soles, or armpits, often with no underlying medical condition.
  - **Secondary (Generalised) Hyperhidrosis:** Caused by underlying conditions such as hyperthyroidism, diabetes, or menopause .

- **Impact:** May lead to discomfort, social embarrassment, and skin infections.

Reduced Sweating (Hypohidrosis or Anhidrosis):

- **Definition:** Inability to sweat adequately in response to heat or exertion.
- **Causes:** Can result from nerve damage (e.g., diabetic neuropathy), skin disorders, or certain medications.

  - **Impact:** Poses a risk of overheating and heatstroke.

Abnormal Smell (Bromhidrosis):

- **Definition:** Unpleasant body odour caused by bacterial breakdown of sweat.

- **Causes:** Often linked to poor hygiene, certain foods, or conditions like trimethylaminuria (6).

FOURTEEN
SLEEP

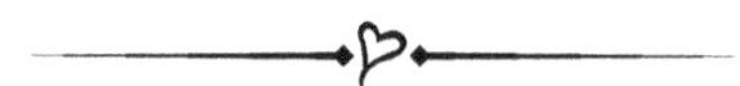

Sleep

Sleep is a vital physiological process that plays a crucial role in maintaining physical, cognitive, and emotional health. It is a state of reduced sensory activity and interaction with the environment, characterised by changes in brain wave activity, muscle relaxation, and metabolic rate.

Normal Sleep

1. **Duration:** Adults typically require 7–9 hours of sleep per night, while children and teenagers require more, depending on age.
2. **Sleep Architecture:** Normal sleep consists of two main phases:

   - **Non-Rapid Eye Movement (NREM) Sleep:** Accounts for about 75–80% of total sleep time, includes light sleep (Stages 1 and 2) and deep sleep (Stage 3).
   - **Rapid Eye Movement (REM) Sleep:** Accounts for 20–25% of sleep and is associated with dreaming and memory consolidation.

2. **Sleep Cycle:** A normal sleep cycle lasts about 90 minutes and repeats 4–6 times per night, alternating between NREM and REM phases.

Abnormal Sleep Patterns

1. **Insomnia:**

   - **Definition:** Difficulty initiating or maintaining sleep, or waking up too early, resulting in daytime impairment.
   - **Causes:** Stress, anxiety, depression, chronic pain, or poor sleep hygiene.

   - **Impact:** Impaired concentration, mood disturbances, and increased risk of chronic diseases.

2. **Hypersomnia:**

   - **Definition:** Excessive sleepiness during the day, even after sufficient nighttime sleep.

- ◦ **Causes:** Sleep apnoea, narcolepsy, or certain medications.

- ◦ **Impact:** Reduced productivity and quality of life.

3. **Sleep Apnoea:**

   - ◦ **Definition:** Interrupted breathing during sleep due to airway obstruction or central nervous system dysfunction.
   - ◦ **Causes:** Obesity, enlarged tonsils, or neurological conditions.

   - ◦ **Impact:** Daytime fatigue, cardiovascular complications, and increased mortality risk.

4. **Circadian Rhythm Disorders:**

   - ◦ **Definition:** Misalignment between the internal body clock and the external environment.

   - ◦ **Causes:** Shift work, jet lag, or delayed sleep phase syndrome.

   - ◦ **Impact:** Impaired sleep quality, mood disturbances, and reduced alertness.

FIFTEEN

MENSES

Menses, or menstruation, is the monthly shedding of the endometrial lining of the uterus, resulting in blood and tissue passing through the vagina. It is a key component of the menstrual cycle, which is regulated by hormonal changes and is vital for reproductive health.

Normal Menstrual Cycle

1. **Duration of Cycle:** The average menstrual cycle lasts 21–35 days, with bleeding typically lasting 2–7 days (1).
2. **Volume of Blood Loss:** Normal blood loss during menstruation ranges from 30–80 mL per cycle (2).
3. **Symptoms:** Mild cramping, breast tenderness, and mood changes may occur but should not significantly interfere with daily activities (3).
4. **Regularity:** Cycles are usually consistent, with predictable intervals, though slight variations are common during adolescence or perimenopause (4).

Abnormal Menstrual Patterns

1. **Heavy Menstrual Bleeding (Menorrhagia):**

   - **Definition:** Excessive bleeding (>80 mL per cycle) or prolonged bleeding (>7 days).

   - **Causes:** Uterine fibroids, adenomyosis, endometrial polyps, or coagulation disorders (5).
   - **Impact:** Can lead to anaemia, fatigue, and reduced quality of life.

1. **Absent or Infrequent Periods (Amenorrhoea and Oligomenorrhoea):**

   - **Definition:** Amenorrhoea refers to the absence of menstruation for three or more cycles, while oligomenorrhoea refers to cycles longer than 35 days.
   - **Causes:** Pregnancy, polycystic ovary syndrome (PCOS), extreme weight loss, or stress .
   - **Impact:** May indicate underlying hormonal imbalances or systemic health issues.

3. **Painful Periods (Dysmenorrhoea):**

   - **Definition:** Severe menstrual cramps that interfere with daily activities.

- ◦ **Causes:** Primary dysmenorrhoea is linked to prostaglandin production, while secondary dysmenorrhoea may result from endometriosis or pelvic inflammatory disease (PID).

4. **Irregular Periods (Metrorrhagia):**

   - ◦ **Definition:** Bleeding at unpredictable intervals, often outside the normal cycle.

   - ◦ **Causes:** Hormonal fluctuations, thyroid dysfunction, or uterine abnormalities.

SIXTEEN

AWARENESS OF OWN ABILITIES

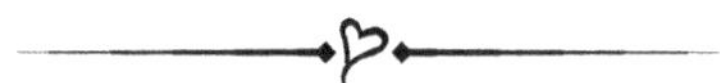

Awareness of one's abilities refers to an individual's understanding and recognition of their strengths, limitations, and potential. This self-awareness is crucial for personal growth, effective decision-making, and adapting to challenges.

Values of Awareness

Well Aware:

- **Definition:** The individual has a clear understanding of their skills, strengths, and areas needing improvement.
- Characteristics:

  - Consistently sets realistic goals based on their abilities.

  - Seeks opportunities to leverage strengths and address weaknesses.

  - Demonstrates confidence without overestimating capabilities.

Somewhat Aware:

- **Definition:** The individual has a partial understanding of their abilities but lacks clarity or consistency.
- Characteristics:

  - May overestimate or underestimate skills in certain areas.

  - Inconsistently utilises strengths or addresses weaknesses.

  - Relies on external feedback to validate abilities.

Not Aware:

- **Definition:** The individual lacks understanding or recognition of their strengths and limitations.

- Characteristics:

  - Struggles to identify personal skills or areas needing growth.

  - Often sets unrealistic goals or avoids challenges due to self-doubt.

  - Shows resistance to feedback or lacks self-reflection.

SEVENTEEN
STRESS COPING LEVELS

"*Stress coping refers to an individual's ability to manage and adapt to stressful situations or challenges effectively. It involves behavioural, emotional, and cognitive strategies to reduce or mitigate the impact of stress on mental and physical health.*"

Levels of Stress Coping

Well Coped:

- **Definition:** The individual effectively manages stress, demonstrating resilience and adaptability in challenging situations.
- Characteristics:

  - Uses healthy coping mechanisms, such as problem-solving, time management, or seeking support.
  - Maintains emotional balance and a positive outlook.

  - Demonstrates physical and mental well-being despite external pressures.

Somewhat Coped:

- **Definition:** The individual manages stress to a certain extent but experiences occasional difficulty in maintaining control.
- Characteristics:

  - Uses a mix of healthy and unhealthy coping strategies, such as procrastination or occasional emotional outbursts.
  - Stress may impact some aspects of daily functioning or relationships.

  - Relies on external help or support to regain balance.

Cannot Cope:

- ◦ **Definition:** The individual struggles to manage stress, leading to significant physical, emotional, or psychological distress.
- ◦ Characteristics:

  - ▪ Avoids or denies problems, often resorting to maladaptive behaviours (e.g., substance abuse, isolation).
  - ▪ Feels overwhelmed, anxious, or helpless in stressful situations.

  - ▪ Experiences frequent disruptions in daily life, such as poor sleep, inability to concentrate, or strained relationships.

EIGHTEEN

PRODUCTIVITY AND FRUITFULNESS

"Productivity and fruitfulness refer to the ability to accomplish tasks, achieve goals, and generate meaningful outcomes in personal and professional settings. These qualities are essential indicators of effectiveness and success in various aspects of life."

Levels of Productivity and Fruitfulness

Good:

- **Definition:** Consistently achieving or exceeding goals with meaningful outcomes.

- Characteristics:

  - Demonstrates efficient time management and prioritisation.

  - Produces high-quality results with minimal effort or waste.

  - Shows innovation, creativity, and problem-solving skills.

Moderate:

- **Definition:** Meeting goals or expectations adequately but with occasional inefficiencies or missed opportunities.
- Characteristics:

  - Demonstrates an average ability to manage tasks and responsibilities.

  - May procrastinate or require external motivation to complete tasks.

  - Achieves results but may lack consistency or innovation.

Bad:

- **Definition:** Consistently failing to achieve goals or produce meaningful outcomes.

- Characteristics:

  - Struggles with time management, organisation, or task prioritisation.

  - Produces low-quality results or fails to meet deadlines.

  - Lacks motivation, focus, or clear direction.

NINETEEN
Past History

"Past history refers to the medical, psychological, or social history of an individual that could provide insights into their current health condition. It plays a critical role in diagnosing, managing, and treating illnesses."

Levels of Relevance

- **Very Relevant:**

  - **Definition:** Past history has a direct and significant connection to the current condition.

  - Examples:

    - History of diabetes in a patient presenting with neuropathy.

    - Previous surgeries related to the organ of complaint.

    - A history of psychiatric illness affecting current mental health.

  - Impact:

    - Crucial for accurate diagnosis and treatment planning.

    - Directly informs decisions on investigations, medication, or interventions.

- **Moderately Relevant:**

  - **Definition:** Past history is related to the condition but has a secondary or indirect influence.
  - Examples:

    - History of smoking in a patient presenting with mild hypertension.

    - Past minor trauma contributing to chronic pain.

- ◦ Impact:

    - ▪ Supports a comprehensive understanding of the patient's condition.

    - ▪ Helps in identifying risk factors or long-term implications.

- **Irrelevant:**

    - ◦ **Definition:** Past history does not have a clear connection to the current condition.

    - ◦ Examples:

        - ▪ A resolved childhood illness with no residual effects in an adult patient.

        - ▪ Unrelated past medical events (e.g., appendectomy in a patient with a migraine).

    - ◦ Impact:

        - ▪ Adds to the overall context but does not directly influence diagnosis or management.

Importance of Assessing Past History

1. **Comprehensive Diagnosis:** Understanding past health issues can reveal underlying causes or contributing factors.
2. **Preventative Care:** Helps in identifying risks for future health problems.

3. **Individualised Treatment:** Guides tailored interventions based on past medical or surgical history.

TWENTY
MENTAL ATTRIBUTES CONTRIBUTING TO ILLNESS

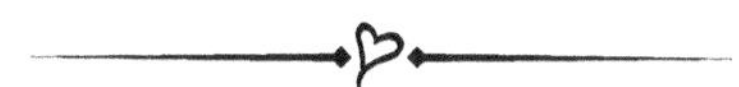

"*Mental attributes such as emotional states, thought patterns, and coping mechanisms can significantly influence physical health and the development or progression of illness. These attributes play a crucial role in the mind-body connection and are often linked to psychosomatic conditions.*"

Categories

1. **Yes (Mental Attributes Contribute to Illness):**

   - **Definition:** Psychological factors that negatively impact health by exacerbating or triggering physical illnesses.
   - Examples of Contributing Attributes:

     - **Chronic Stress:** Prolonged stress can lead to hormonal imbalances, suppressed immunity, and increased risk of cardiovascular diseases.
     - **Anxiety and Depression:** Persistent negative emotions may contribute to gastrointestinal disorders, chronic pain, or weakened immune response.
     - **Poor Coping Mechanisms:** Behaviours like substance abuse or avoidance can worsen conditions such as hypertension or diabetes.

2. No (Mental Attributes Do Not Contribute to Illness):

   - **Definition:** Psychological factors are not significant contributors to illness in certain conditions, with primary causation being genetic, infectious, or environmental.
   - Examples:

     - Genetic disorders (e.g., cystic fibrosis).

     - Acute infectious diseases (e.g., malaria).

     - Trauma-related conditions without significant psychological involvement.

TWENTY-ONE
LEVELS ON EMOTIONAL SCALE

"The emotional scale categorises emotions into three levels based on their intensity and impact on mental and physical well-being. Understanding and managing these emotions is crucial for maintaining emotional intelligence and overall health."

Level 1: Positive Emotions

- **Emotions:** Joy, Love, Optimism, Hopefulness.

- Characteristics:

  - Associated with feelings of happiness, contentment, and motivation.

  - Promote resilience, creativity, and social bonding.

  - Positively impact physical health by reducing stress hormones and improving immune function.

- Impact:

  - Enhances problem-solving abilities and decision-making.

  - Strengthens interpersonal relationships and self-esteem .

Level 2: Moderate Emotions

- **Emotions:** Doubt, Frustration, Anxiety.

- Characteristics:

  - Represent a middle ground where emotions fluctuate based on external circumstances.

- ○ Can act as a driving force to resolve uncertainties or improve performance.

- ○ When prolonged, may lead to stress or hinder productivity.

- Impact:

  - ○ Encourages self-reflection and adaptability.

  - ○ If unmanaged, can escalate to negative emotions or impair decision-making.

Level 3: Negative Emotions

- **Emotions:** Anger, Grief, Fear, Despair, Shame, Guilt.

- Characteristics:

  - ○ Associated with stress, helplessness, or regret.

  - ○ Trigger the "fight or flight" response, increasing cortisol levels.

  - ○ Prolonged exposure can lead to mental health issues like depression, anxiety, or burnout.

- Impact:

  - ○ Impairs judgment, social relationships, and overall well-being.

  - ○ Requires active coping strategies to prevent long-term effects.

TWENTY-TWO
FAMILY HISTORY

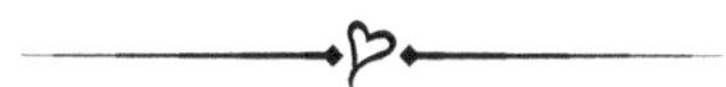

"Family history refers to the medical conditions, genetic disorders, or chronic diseases present in an individual's immediate or extended family. It provides valuable insights into hereditary risks and predispositions for certain health conditions."

Levels of Relevance

1. **Very Relevant:**

   - **Definition:** Family history has a direct and significant connection to the individual's current or potential health condition.
   - Examples:

     - A family history of diabetes in a patient with unexplained hyperglycaemia.

     - Genetic conditions like BRCA mutations for breast or ovarian cancer risk.

     - Cardiovascular diseases in close relatives influencing a patient's risk profile.

   - Impact:

     - Crucial for early diagnosis, preventative measures, and personalised treatment plans.
     - Directly influences decisions on screening, lifestyle modifications, or interventions (1).

2. Moderately Relevant:

   - **Definition:** Family history has an indirect or partial influence on the individual's health condition.
   - Examples:

     - A distant relative with asthma in a patient with mild respiratory symptoms.

     - Family history of hypertension contributing to a moderate risk in a patient with a sedentary lifestyle.

- Impact:

  - Helps identify potential risks or underlying genetic predispositions.

  - Supports comprehensive risk assessments (2).

1. Irrelevant:

   - **Definition:** Family history has no apparent connection to the individual's current health condition or risk factors.
   - Examples:

     - A family history of gastrointestinal disorders in a patient presenting with migraines.

Family history of unrelated conditions in a patient with no overlapping symptoms

TWENTY-THREE
TREATMENT HISTORY

"Treatment history refers to the record of past medical interventions, including medications, surgeries, therapies, or alternative treatments. It provides valuable context for understanding the progression of an individual's health condition and planning future care."

Levels of Relevance

Very Relevant:

- **Definition:** Past treatments have a direct and significant impact on the individual's current condition or influence the choice of ongoing management.
- Examples:

  - Previous use of antibiotics in a patient with recurrent infections to avoid resistance issues.
  - History of chemotherapy or radiotherapy affecting current symptoms or treatment options.
  - Past surgical interventions altering anatomy or physiology, such as gastrointestinal surgeries.

- Impact:

  - Guides the selection of safe and effective treatment options.

  - Provides insights into treatment effectiveness, side effects, or complications .

Moderately Relevant:

- **Definition:** Past treatments are somewhat related to the current condition but have limited influence on immediate care decisions.
- Examples:

  - History of physical therapy for joint pain in a patient presenting with a new injury.
  - Use of over-the-counter supplements in a patient with chronic fatigue.

- Impact:

- Helps provide a broader context for understanding the patient's medical history.

- May assist in identifying long-term patterns or risks.

Irrelevant:

- **Definition:** Past treatments have no apparent connection to the individual's current condition or care plan.
- Examples:

  - A history of childhood immunisations in a patient presenting with an unrelated condition.
  - Previous treatment for minor, resolved illnesses like the common cold.

TWENTY-FOUR
PERSONAL HISTORY

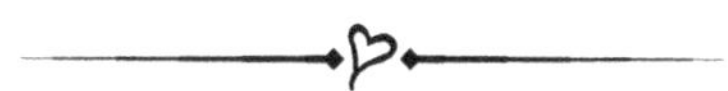

"Personal history encompasses a broad range of personal details such as upbringing, education, occupation, vaccination status, dietary habits, sexual health, and general appearance. This information helps in understanding the patient's background, lifestyle, and social determinants of health."

Levels of Relevance

1. **Very Relevant:**

   - **Definition:** Aspects of personal history that have a direct and significant impact on the patient's current health condition or treatment plan.
   - Examples:

     - **Born and Brought Up:** Geographic origin relevant to endemic diseases (e.g., malaria, tuberculosis).
     - **Dietary Habits:** Nutritional deficiencies or high-risk diets contributing to conditions like obesity or diabetes.
     - **Sexual Functions:** History of sexually transmitted infections or issues affecting reproductive health.
     - **General Appearance:** Observations like pallor, jaundice, or cachexia indicating systemic diseases.

   - Impact:

     - Provides essential insights for diagnosis and management.

     - Directly influences preventive and therapeutic interventions (1).

1. Moderately Relevant:

   - **Definition:** Aspects of personal history that provide additional context but are not directly linked to the current condition.
   - Examples:

     - **Education and Occupation:** Impact on health literacy or exposure to occupational hazards.

- **Vaccination History:** General immunity or risk factors for vaccine- preventable diseases.

  - Impact:

    - Supports a holistic understanding of the patient's background.

    - Assists in tailoring health education or preventive measures (2).

3. Irrelevant:

   - **Definition:** Aspects of personal history unrelated to the current health issue or treatment plan.
   - Examples:

     - **Born and Brought Up:** Geographic origin with no link to the presenting condition.
     - **Education or Occupation:** Information that does not affect health risks or management.

   - Impact:

     - Provides general background but does not contribute to immediate care decisions (3).

References:

1. Marmot M, Allen J, Bell R, Bloomer E, Goldblatt P. WHO European review of social determinants of health and the health divide. Lancet. 2012;380(9846):1011–29. doi:10.1016/S0140-6736(12)61228-8.
2. Adler NE, Newman K. Socioeconomic disparities in health: Pathways and policies. Health Aff. 2002;21(2):60–76. doi:10.1377/hlthaff.21.60.
3. Wilkinson RG, Marmot MG, editors. Social determinants of health: The solid facts. 2nd ed. Copenhagen: World Health Organization; 200

TWENTY-FIVE
INTENSITY

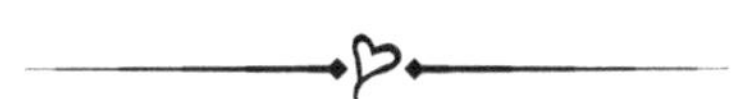

Trivial

- **Definition:** Minimal symptoms with negligible impact on daily life and no significant organ dysfunction.
- **Examples:** Controlled mild hypertension, minor skin conditions like mild acne.

Mild

- **Definition:** Symptoms are present but do not significantly interfere with daily activities; minimal organ involvement.
- **Examples:** Early-stage type 2 diabetes with controlled blood glucose levels, mild osteoarthritis with occasional discomfort.

Moderate

- **Definition:** Symptoms moderately impair daily functioning, with noticeable organ involvement.
- **Examples:** Moderate chronic kidney disease (CKD) with declining renal function, COPD with reduced lung capacity (FEV1 50–80%).

Severe

- **Definition:** Symptoms significantly impair quality of life, with advanced organ involvement affecting functionality.
- **Examples:** Azoospermia impacting fertility, advanced heart failure with marked functional limitations.

Very Severe

- **Definition:** Life-threatening symptoms with profound systemic effects and extensive organ involvement.
- **Examples:** End-stage renal disease requiring dialysis, terminal cancer with widespread metastasis.

TWENTY-SIX
DURATION OF DISEASE

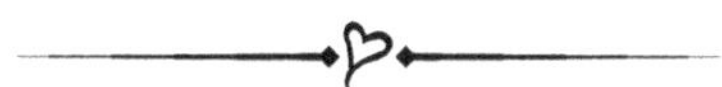

"*The duration of a disease refers to the length of time the condition has persisted, providing critical insights into its progression and management requirements.*"

Duration Categories with Definitions

Less than 10 days:

- **Definition:** Acute conditions that resolve within 10 days.

- **Examples:** Common cold, mild viral infections.

11 days to 1 month:

- **Definition:** Subacute conditions lasting longer than 10 days but less than a month.

- **Examples:** Acute bronchitis, recovery phase of minor injuries.

1 month to 6 months:

- **Definition:** Prolonged conditions lasting up to 6 months, often requiring ongoing care.

- **Examples:** Subacute bacterial endocarditis, prolonged viral illnesses.

6 months to 1 year:

- **Definition:** Conditions persisting beyond 6 months but not yet considered chronic.

- **Examples:** Hepatitis B infections under observation, certain post-surgical recovery phases.

1 year to 3 years:

- **Definition:** Long-standing conditions often managed as chronic diseases.

- ◦ **Examples:** Controlled diabetes diagnosed within the last three years, newly diagnosed rheumatoid arthritis.

More than 3 years:

- ◦ **Definition:** Chronic or long-term conditions persisting for over three years.

- ◦ **Examples:** Long-standing hypertension, COPD, or chronic kidney disease.

TWENTY-SEVEN
DREADFULNESS

Levels of Dreadfulness

1. **Reversible without Medication:**

   - **Definition:** Conditions where functional changes resolve naturally without the need for medical intervention.
   - **Examples:** Mild dehydration, muscle soreness from exercise.

1. Gross Functional Disturbances:

   - **Definition:** Significant functional impairments without evident pathological changes.

   - **Examples:** Acute stress-induced hypertension, functional dyspepsia.

3. Grade 1 Pathological Changes:

   - **Definition:** Initial pathological changes that may require treatment or observation but are manageable.
   - **Examples:** Fatty liver without inflammation, early stages of anaemia.

4. Grade 2 Pathological Changes:

   - **Definition:** Established pathology requiring mandatory treatment, observation, or lifestyle modifications.
   - **Examples:** Moderate diabetic neuropathy, hypertension with target organ involvement.

5. Pathology with Complications:

   - **Definition:** Pathological changes with complications affecting multiple systems or organ functions.
   - **Examples:** Diabetes with retinopathy, chronic kidney disease with anaemia.

Irreversible Pathological Changes:

- ◦ **Definition:** Permanent damage to organs or systems where rehabilitation is the only intervention.
- ◦ **Examples:** End-stage renal disease, myocardial infarction with significant cardiac dysfunction.

TWENTY-EIGHT
Extent of Disease

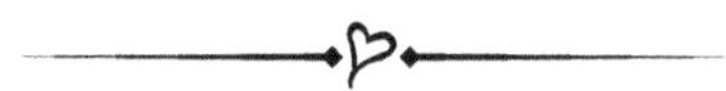

"The extent of disease defines the level of organ involvement, focusing on whether the changes are benign, pathological, or uncontrollable. The classification includes specific attention to vital organs, which are defined as organs whose damage affects their structure and function significantly."

Levels of Extent

Affects Superficial Organ - Benign Affection:

- **Definition:** Disease limited to a single superficial organ with non-threatening and manageable changes.
- **Examples:** Mild dermatitis, superficial abscess.

Affects Internal Organ - Benign Affection:

- **Definition:** Disease limited to a single internal organ, causing manageable changes without structural or functional compromise.
- **Examples:** Mild gastritis, simple hepatic cyst.

Pathological or Uncontrollable Changes in Internal or Superficial Organs:

- **Definition:** Disease involving superficial or internal organs with pathological or uncontrollable changes requiring intervention.
- **Examples:** Severe eczema with infection, peptic ulcer disease with bleeding.

Progressive Pathological or Uncontrollable Changes in Internal or Superficial Organs:

- **Definition:** Disease causing progressive and severe pathological or uncontrollable changes in superficial or internal organs.
- **Examples:** Advanced liver fibrosis, inflammatory bowel disease with complications.

Affects Vital Organs (Excludes Renal Calculi):

- **Definition:** Disease impacting vital organs (e.g., heart, brain, lungs, liver) where damage affects their structure and function significantly. Renal calculi are excluded as they do not directly impair organ survival functions.
- **Examples:** Acute heart failure, chronic obstructive pulmonary disease with severe respiratory impairment.

Multi-System Disease and Metastasis:

- **Definition:** Disease involving multiple organ systems or systemic spread (metastasis). "Metastasis" here refers to the spread of any uncontrollable condition, not limited to cancer.
- **Examples:** Advanced systemic lupus erythematosus with multi-organ involvement, widespread sepsis.

TWENTY-NINE
NATURE OF CHRONIC DISEASE

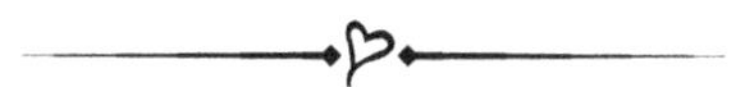

"The nature of chronic disease describes its progression, management requirements, and potential outcomes. Chronic diseases often require long-term care and are classified based on their ability to resolve, the need for medical intervention, and their potential complications or impact."

Levels of Nature of Chronic Disease

Self-Limiting, No Intervention Needed:

- **Definition:** Conditions that stabilise or resolve naturally with minimal lifestyle adjustments.
- **Examples:** Mild non-alcoholic fatty liver disease, prehypertension managed with diet and exercise.

Self-Limiting with Complications:

- **Definition:** Conditions that stabilise but may lead to complications if proper lifestyle modifications or care are neglected.
- **Examples:** Pre-diabetes with potential progression to type 2 diabetes if unmanaged.

Self-Limiting Which Require Immediate Attention:

- **Definition:** Conditions that can stabilise naturally but require immediate intervention to prevent severe complications.
- **Examples:** Acute mild asthma attacks are managed with short-term bronchodilators.

Non-Self-Limiting:

- **Definition:** Conditions requiring continuous medical management, as they cannot stabilise or resolve on their own.
- **Examples:** Chronic obstructive pulmonary disease (COPD), hypertension.

Non-Self-Limiting with Complications:

- **Definition:** Conditions that require medical intervention and present with complications impacting one or more organ systems.

- **Examples:** Type 2 diabetes with retinopathy, chronic kidney disease with anaemia.

Causes Permanent Deterioration and Deformity:

- **Definition:** Chronic diseases leading to structural or functional damage, resulting in long-term disability or deformity.

- **Examples:** Type 2 diabetes with retinopathy, chronic kidney disease with anaemia.

THIRTY

Applications of the Scoring System

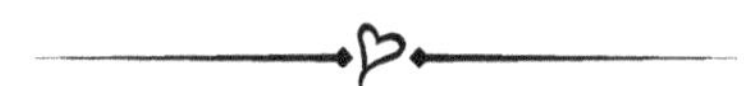

"*The Hidden Protocol scoring system offers wide-ranging applications in homoeopathic practice, extending beyond case evaluation. It serves as a tool for improving clinical accuracy, enhancing patient communication, streamlining research, and integrating technology for advanced homoeopathic care. This section explores the practical applications of the scoring system in various domains.*"

1. Clinical Practice

- 1.1 Case Analysis and Diagnosis

  - Objective Evaluation: The scoring system translates subjective symptoms into measurable data, helping practitioners identify key issues and prioritise them.
  - Example: A high emotional score combined with moderate disease scores suggests a focus on emotional management in treatment.

- 1.2 Remedy Selection

  - Guided Prescription: The scores highlight the dominant aspects of a case, aiding in remedy selection tailored to the patient's needs.
  - Example: Remedies addressing grief or anxiety might be prioritised for a high emotional score.

- 1.3 Prognosis

  - Predictive Insights: The system estimates curability and treatment duration based on disease and health scores.
  - Example: Cases with lower HP scores are likely to recover faster with proper intervention.

- 1.4 Treatment Monitoring

  - Dynamic Scoring: Follow-up evaluations allow practitioners to track progress and adjust treatment strategies.
  - Example: A declining disease score over time confirms treatment efficacy.

2. Patient Engagement

- 2.1 Communication

- ◦ Transparent Discussions: The scoring system provides a visual and numeric representation of the patient's condition, fostering trust and understanding.
- ◦ Example: Sharing a curability chart helps patients comprehend their health trajectory.

- **2.2 Expectation Management**

  - ◦ Realistic Goals: Scores guide practitioners in setting achievable outcomes, reducing patient frustration.
  - ◦ Example: A patient with a high disease score may be advised to expect gradual progress.

- **2.3 Empowerment**

  - ◦ Active Participation: Patients can understand their health status better and take an active role in their treatment.
  - ◦ Example: Providing personalised lifestyle recommendations based on their scores.

3. Research and Education

- **3.1 Data Collection**

  - ◦ Case Databases: The scoring system creates a structured database for analysing treatment outcomes and remedy efficacy.
  - ◦ Example: Aggregated data can reveal trends in miasmatic influences or remedy responses.

- **3.2 Evidence Generation**

  - ◦ Clinical Validation: Standardised scoring allows for rigorous testing of homoeopathic principles and practices.
  - ◦ Example: Comparing outcomes across cases with similar HP scores to validate a treatment protocol.

- **3.3 Training Tool**

  - ◦ Educational Resource: The scoring system can be incorporated into homoeopathic curricula, training students in systematic case analysis.
  - ◦ Example: Simulated cases scored by students to enhance diagnostic skills.

4. Integration with Technology

- **4.1 Digital Tools**

  - ◦ Software Integration: The scoring system can be incorporated into electronic medical record systems and homoeopathic apps for streamlined practice.
  - ◦ Example: Automated scoring calculators linked to patient profiles.

- **4.2 AI and Machine Learning**

  - ◦ Predictive Models: Aggregated data can train AI models to predict outcomes or suggest remedies based on case scores.
  - ◦ Example: AI recommending high-probability remedies for specific HP score ranges.

- 4.3 Remote Consultations

  - Telemedicine: Scoring simplifies remote evaluations by standardising case details.
  - Example: Patients filling out scoring forms before virtual consultations.

5. Policy and Standardisation

- 5.1 Practice Guidelines

  - Protocol Development: The system lays the groundwork for standardised treatment guidelines in homoeopathy.
  - Example: Defining clear steps for managing Level 4 cases across practices.

- 5.2 Certification

  - Professional Accreditation: Scoring proficiency can become a benchmark for certifying homoeopaths.
  - Example: Practitioners scoring accurately on simulated cases receive advanced certifications.

- 5.3 Global Standardisation

  - Uniform Practice: By adopting the scoring system, homoeopaths worldwide can align their practices, improving consistency and collaboration.
  - Example: International conferences analysing cross-regional data trends.

6. Advanced Applications

- 6.1 Integrative Medicine

  - Collaboration with Modern Medicine: The scoring system bridges homoeopathy with other disciplines by presenting measurable health data.
  - Example: Shared scoring criteria for evaluating chronic conditions in integrative clinics.

- 6.2 Public Health

  - Epidemiological Studies: Large-scale scoring data can provide insights into disease prevalence and treatment outcomes.
  - Example: Analysing miasmatic influences in endemic regions.

- 6.3 Personalised Medicine

  - Custom Protocols: Scores enable the creation of highly individualised treatment plans.
  - Example: Tailoring remedies and lifestyle modifications based on a patient's holistic profile.

"The Hidden Protocol scoring system is more than a diagnostic tool; it is a transformative framework for enhancing every aspect of homoeopathic practice. Its applications in clinical practice, patient engagement, research, technology integration, and policy development ensure its pivotal role in the modernisation of homoeopathy."

THIRTY-ONE

A Standardised Plan of Treatment - The Hidden Protocol in Action

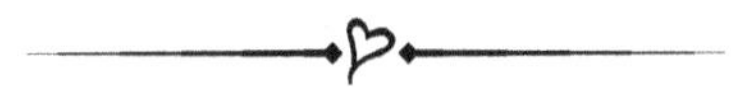

Step 1: Evaluating the Patient

Before any treatment begins, the foundation lies in accurately evaluating the patient using the protocol's scoring system.
Action:

- Assign scores across parameters like General Health, Mental and Emotional States, Disease Characteristics, and Historical Factors.

Outcome:

- A comprehensive and objective assessment of the patient's condition.

Step 2: Interpreting the Holistic Potential (HP) Score

The HP Score acts as the practitioner's compass, directing the course of treatment.
Action:

- Combine the Health and Disease scores to derive the HP Score.

Outcome:

- The HP Score categorises the patient into one of six levels, each with a specific plan of treatment.

The Levels of Treatment: A Dynamic Blueprint

Each HP Score range represents a distinct level of treatment complexity. Let's explore the six levels, adding a touch of practical insight and wisdom from Dr P. Radhakrishnan's decades of experience

Level 1: Simple Case (HP Score: 6–10)

"Every patient is unique, but not every case needs complexity. Simplicity often holds the key to swift recovery."
— Dr P. Radhakrishnan

- Characteristics:

  ◦ Mild conditions are easily manageable with a single remedy.

- Plan of Treatment:

  ◦ Symptom similarity alone is sufficient.
  ◦ Focus on remedies based on presenting complaints and altered generals.

- Follow-Up:

  ◦ Routine check-ups to monitor progress.

- Prognosis:

  ◦ High curability with minimal intervention.

Level 2: Careful Case (HP Score: 11–15)

""Careful observation and subtle intervention define the success of these cases."
— Dr P. Radhakrishnan"

Characteristics:

- Conditions requiring both symptom analysis and basic pathology insights.

Plan of Treatment:

- Combine remedies addressing symptoms and underlying pathology.
- Incorporate auxiliary measures like diet modification.

Follow-Up:

- Monitor for emerging complications.

Prognosis:

- Good recovery potential with moderate intervention.

Level 3: Cautious Case (HP Score: 16–20)

"These cases demand vigilance, skill, and a deep understanding of the patient's inner terrain."
– Dr P. Radhakrishnan

- **Characteristics**:

  ○ Moderate severity, requiring a mix of symptom, pathology, and miasmatic analysis.

- **Plan of Treatment**:

○ Miasmatic remedies play a pivotal role alongside symptomatic treatment and pathological assessment.
  ○ Lifestyle modifications are crucial.

- **Follow-Up**:

  ○ Comprehensive monitoring to ensure gradual progress.

- **Prognosis**:

  ○ Recovery depends on adherence to the plan and close observation.

Level 4: Extra Care Case (HP Score: 21–25)

"Prognosis becomes a critical component here—knowing when to act and when to wait is the hallmark of expertise."
– Dr P. Radhakrishnan

Characteristics:

- Complex cases where symptoms, pathology, and prognosis intertwine.

Plan of Treatment:

- Surgical options may be needed for homoeopathic remedies.
- Advanced pathological and miasmatic remedies are essential.

Follow-Up:

- Frequent visits to adapt the treatment as required.
- The chance of getting complicated is higher, so frequent investigations and thorough prognostic assessments are mandatory

Prognosis:

- Progress may be slower, requiring both patience and precision.

Level 5: Expert Case (HP Score: 26–30)

"These cases test a homoeopath's mettle. It's where experience meets intuition and science."
— Dr P. Radhakrishnan

Characteristics:

- Severe conditions with significant complexity.

Plan of Treatment:

- Precision in similimum selection is non-negotiable. The selection of similimum using the method of triangles, where the accurate similimum is acquired.
- Prognostic assessments guide the course of action.
- Surgery may be necessary as an adjunct.

Follow-Up:

- Intensive and frequent, with a focus on nuanced adjustments.

Prognosis:

- Complex but achievable with the right approach.

Level 6: Palliative Case (HP Score: 31–36)

"When cure is unattainable, compassion becomes the cornerstone of treatment."
– Dr P. Radhakrishnan

Characteristics:

- Conditions beyond curative possibilities, focusing on quality of life.

Plan of Treatment:

- Palliative remedies to alleviate suffering and enhance well-being.
  - Psychological and emotional support is paramount.
- Medicines covering the symptoms and pathology is more suited.

Follow-Up:

- Regular reviews to adjust remedies and ensure comfort.

Prognosis:

- Focused on maintaining dignity and relief.

THIRTY-TWO

INDICES OF THE HIDDEN PROTOCOL – THE CORNERSTONES OF PRECISION IN HOMOEOPATHY

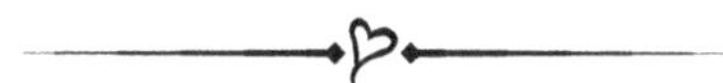

<u>Revolutionising Homoeopathy with Data-Driven Insights</u>

In the ever-evolving field of homoeopathy, clarity and precision in treatment planning remain paramount. The Hidden Protocol introduces a groundbreaking set of indices that quantify essential aspects of patient evaluation, bridging the gap between subjective interpretation and objective decision-making. These indices— Disease Severity Index, Case Score, and Curability Index—form the backbone of this innovative tool, ensuring practitioners make informed choices with every case.

This visionary framework was developed by Dr P. Nidheesh, an internationally acclaimed homoeopath, philosopher, hypnotherapist, and researcher. Drawing from decades of experience and the invaluable teachings of his father, Dr P. Radhakrishnan, a pioneer in homoeopathy, Dr Nidheesh crafted this tool as an act of benevolence, aimed at empowering homoeopaths worldwide. By observing and systematising his father's unparalleled treatment methods, Dr Nidheesh has given the homoeopathic community a legacy of knowledge.

Curability Index (CI)

"The ultimate indicator of the chance of disease resolution."

Definition:

- The Curability Index estimates the percentage chance of curing the disease. It provides a direct, actionable metric for both practitioners and patients.

How It's Calculated:

The CI is derived by comparing:

- Health Scores: Resilience and vitality.
- Disease Scores: Extent, severity, and chronicity of the disease.

Implications:

- ***High CI (Above 75%):***

  ○ Indicates a strong likelihood of recovery with homoeopathic treatment alone.

- ***Moderate CI (50–75%):***

  ○ Suggests curative potential, but treatment may require longer durations or adjunctive therapies.

- ***Low CI (Below 50%):***

  ○ Highlights poor curability; treatment focuses on managing symptoms and improving quality of life.

Purpose in Practice:

The CI provides practitioners with an evidence-based measure to counsel patients and plan interventions.

Empowering Homoeopaths with Clarity and Confidence

The indices of The Hidden Protocol are a testament to the evolution of homoeopathy. By quantifying the abstract, they bring consistency and reliability to treatment planning. From gauging curability to assessing disease severity, these indices empower homoeopaths to make informed, impactful decisions.

THIRTY-THREE
DETAILED METHOD OF CALCULATION

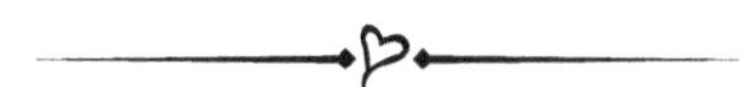

General Parameters include the following six items:

- Appetite
- Thirst
- Stool
- Urine
- Sweat
- Sleep
- (Menses – Optional, used only if applicable)

Scoring Rules
For each item:

- If the parameter is normal, it is scored as 0 points.
- If the parameter is abnormal (meaning deviation from healthy function), it is scored as 0.5 points.

Menses field special rule:

- If the patient is male, climacteric (post-menopausal), or a small girl, the Menses parameter is automatically marked as 'Not Applicable' and scored 0 points.
- If Menses is applicable, it follows the same rule:
- Normal menstrual cycle = 0 points
- Abnormal menstrual cycle (irregularities) = 0.5 points.

Step-by-Step Calculation
Start with Appetite:

- If the child eats regularly and normally → 0 points.
- If reduced appetite (loss of hunger) or excessive eating → 0.5 points.

Next, Thirst:

- If thirst is appropriate to weather and activity → 0 points.
- If there is increased thirst (e.g., frequent drinking) or decreased thirst → 0.5 points.

Then, Stool:

- If regular bowel movement (once a day or as per normal habits) → 0 points.
- If constipation (less than 3 times a week) or diarrhoea (more than 3 times a day) → 0.5 points.

Then, Urine:

- If normal urination without pain, normal colour → 0 points.
- If painful urination, blood in urine, frequent urge, burning sensation → 0.5 points.

Then, Sweat:

- If normal sweating depending on temperature, activity → 0 points.
- If excessive sweating (profuse, night sweats) or very little sweating → 0.5 points.

Then, Sleep:

- If the child sleeps peacefully, regular time → 0 points.
- If trouble falling asleep, frequent waking, disturbed sleep → 0.5 points.

Finally, Menses:

- If not applicable (male, small child, or menopause) → 0 points.
- If normal periods → 0 points.
- If irregular periods (early, delayed, scanty, profuse) → 0.5 points.

After evaluating all seven fields:

- Add up the points from Appetite + Thirst + Stool + Urine + Sweat + Sleep (+ Menses if applicable).
- This gives the General Parameters Subtotal.

Mental Generals section includes three key items:

- Awareness of Abilities
- Stress Coping Level
- Productivity and Fruitfulness

Scoring Rules
For each Mental General parameter:

- Best Condition (Healthy): 0 points
- Moderate Disturbance: 1 point
- Severe Disturbance: 2 points

Thus, the worse the mental function, the higher the score assigned.
Step-by-Step Calculation
Awareness of Abilities:

- If the patient is well aware of their strengths and capabilities → 0 points.
- If the patient is only somewhat aware (partial self-understanding) → 1 point.
- If the patient is not aware of their abilities at all (low self-confidence, confusion about self) → 2 points.

ᗰᗰᗰ

Stress Coping Level:

- If the patient copes well with stress and recovers from pressure easily → 0 points.
- If the patient copes somewhat (partial resilience, occasional breakdowns) → 1 point.
- If the patient cannot cope with stress (frequent emotional breakdowns, panic, despair) → 2 points.

ᗰᗰᗰ

Productivity and Fruitfulness:

- If the patient is highly productive (good school performance, work output, creativity, achievements) → 0 points.
- If the patient is moderately productive (average output, sometimes good sometimes poor) → 1 point.
- If the patient is unproductive (failure to deliver results, chronic lack of performance) → 2 points.

ᗰᗰᗰ

After evaluating all three fields:
Add up the points from Awareness of Abilities + Stress Coping Level + Productivity.
Example:

- Awareness: Well Aware → 0 points
- Stress Coping: Somewhat Coped → 1 point
- Productivity: Moderate → 1 point

Mental Generals subtotal = 0 + 1 + 1 = 2 points

Important Points to Remember

- Perfect mental health gives 0 points in total for Mental Generals.
- Moderate problems cause the Mental Generals subtotal to rise to 2–3 points.
- Severe mental dysfunction causes higher scores (up to 6 points maximum from Mental Generals alone).
- This subtotal becomes part of the overall Health Sum which influences the Health Score.

Emotional Attributes section includes two important items:

- Mental Attributes Contributing to Illness
- Level on Emotional Scale

Scoring Rules
Each item has fixed scoring:
Mental Attributes Contributing to Illness:

- If No → 0 points
- If Yes → 2 points

ᛈᛈᛈ

Level on Emotional Scale:

- Level 1 (Positive Emotions: Joy, Love, Optimism, Hopefulness) → 0 points
- Level 2 (Moderate Negative Emotions: Frustration, Anxiety, Doubt) → 1 point
- Level 3 (Severe Negative Emotions: Anger, Grief, Fear, Despair) → 2 points

Thus, more emotional disturbance = higher score.

ᛈᛈᛈ

Step-by-Step Calculation
Mental Attributes Contributing to Illness:

- If the patient's mental/emotional issues are not significantly contributing to their physical illness → 0 points.
- If emotional disturbances are definitely contributing to illness aggravation or causation → 2 points.

Level on Emotional Scale:

- If the patient mainly experiences positive emotions, maintaining optimism and hope → 0 points.
- If the patient shows moderate negative emotions, such as frequent frustration, mild anxiety, self-doubt → 1 point.
- If the patient experiences severe negative emotions, such as anger outbursts, deep grief, chronic fear, despair → 2 points.

After evaluating both fields:

- Add up the points from Mental Attributes Contributing to Illness + Emotional Scale.

Example:

- Mental Attributes Contributing to Illness: Yes → 2 points
- Emotional Level: Moderate Negative Emotions → 1 point
- Emotional Attributes subtotal = 2 + 1 = 3 points

Important Points to Remember

- A completely positive and stable emotional health will add 0 points to the Health Sum.
- Minor emotional disturbances can add 1–3 points.
- Major emotional disturbances will add up to 4 points maximum in Emotional Attributes.
- Emotional instability has a direct influence on the curability and constitutional stability of the patient.
- Emotional Attributes subtotal becomes part of the full Health Sum.

ᛈᛈᛈ

History section includes four important items:

- Past History
- Family History
- Treatment History (Continuing Treatments)
- Personal History (Habits, Appearance, Stress, etc.)

ᚦᚦᚦ

Scoring Rules

- For each History parameter:
- No Significant History → 0 points
- Moderate History → 1 point
- Very Strong History → 2 points

Thus, the more severe or impactful the historical health issues, the higher the score assigned.

ᚦᚦᚦ

Step-by-Step Calculation
Past History:

- If there is no significant medical past (no major diseases, accidents, surgeries) → 0 points.
- If there is a moderate past history (e.g., past infections, minor surgeries, repeated illnesses) → 1 point.
- If there is a very strong past history (e.g., history of major diseases like tuberculosis, cancer, major surgeries, severe infections) → 2 points.

ᚦᚦᚦ

Family History:

- If there is no family history of major illnesses → 0 points.
- If there is a moderate family history (e.g., diabetes, hypertension in immediate relatives) → 1 point.
- If there is a very strong family history (e.g., strong genetic diseases, cancer, autoimmune disorders across multiple generations) → 2 points.

ᚦᚦᚦ

Treatment History (Continuing Treatments also included):

- If there is no ongoing treatment at present → 0 points.
- If the patient is under moderate treatment (e.g., taking medicines for minor conditions) → 1 point.
- If there is very strong or aggressive ongoing treatment (e.g., chemotherapy, immunosuppressants, chronic steroid use) → 2 points.

ᚦᚦᚦ

Personal History:

- If the patient has no significant lifestyle concerns (healthy habits, good appearance, low stress) → 0 points.
- If there are moderate concerns (e.g., mild stress, irregular habits, minor appearance issues) → 1 point.
- If there are very strong concerns (e.g., substance abuse, extreme stress levels, marked unhealthy lifestyle) → 2 points.

ᚦᚦᚦ

After evaluating all four fields:

Add up the points from Past History + Family History + Treatment History + Personal History.

ᚦᚦᚦ

Example:

- Past History: Very Strong → 2 points
- Family History: Moderate → 1 point
- Treatment History: No History → 0 points
- Personal History: Moderate → 1 point

History subtotal = 2 + 1 + 0 + 1 = 4 points

ᚦᚦᚦ

Important Points to Remember

- History section can contribute a maximum of 8 points (2 × 4 fields).
- Minor past and family history issues will add only 1–2 points.
- Major health burdens or genetic risks will add higher values.
- History subtotal becomes an essential part of the full Health Sum, indicating how deeply rooted the disease susceptibility is.

ᚦᚦᚦ

Disease Parameters include five main items:

- Intensity
- Duration of Presenting Complaint
- Dreadfulness of Disease
- Extent of Disease
- Nature of Disease

ᚦᚦᚦ

Scoring Rules

- Each Disease Parameter is scored directly, based on severity, with predefined levels:
- Mildest condition gets the lowest score (1 point).
- Most severe or advanced condition gets the highest score (6 points).
- Each parameter must be individually evaluated and the score assigned according to clinical judgment and investigation findings.

ᚦᚦᚦ

Step-by-Step Calculation
Intensity (Severity of current complaint):

- 1 point → Trivial complaints (e.g., mild cold, minor bruises)
- 2 points → Mild complaints (e.g., mild gastritis, skin rash)
- 3 points → Moderate complaints (e.g., asthma attacks, moderate infections)
- 4 points → Severe complaints (e.g., pneumonia, severe arthritis)
- 5 points → Very severe (e.g., life-threatening conditions needing hospital care)
- 6 points → Life-threatening emergencies (e.g., organ failure, septic shock)

ᚦᚦᚦ

Duration of Presenting Complaint (How long the problem has lasted):

- 1 point → Less than 10 days
- 2 points → 11 days to 1 month
- 3 points → 1–6 months
- 4 points → 6 months to 1 year
- 5 points → 1–3 years
- 6 points → More than 3 years

ᚦᚦᚦ

Dreadfulness of Disease (The pathological seriousness of the disease):

- 1 point → Reversible without medication
- 2 points → Gross functional disturbances (functional problems without major tissue changes)
- 3 points → Grade 1 pathological changes (early tissue damage)
- 4 points → Grade 2 pathological changes (advanced tissue destruction)
- 5 points → Pathology with complications (e.g., kidney failure in diabetes)
- 6 points → Irreversible pathological changes (permanent damage, e.g., cirrhosis)

ÞÞÞ

Extent of Disease (How widely the disease has affected the body):

- 1 point → Superficial organ benign affection (e.g., skin conditions, external wounds)
- 2 points → Internal organ benign affection (e.g., mild liver swelling)
- 3 points → Malignant changes in internal or superficial organs (e.g., localised cancer)
- 4 points → Malignant changes affecting multiple internal organs
- 5 points → Affects vital organs (e.g., heart, brain, kidneys)
- 6 points → Multi-system diseases or metastasis (e.g., widespread cancer)

ÞÞÞ

Nature of Disease (Is it self-resolving or destructive?):

- 1 point → Self-limiting disease needing no intervention (e.g., common cold)
- 2 points → Self-limiting but with complications (e.g., dengue fever leading to bleeding)
- 3 points → Requires immediate attention (e.g., appendicitis)
- 4 points → Non-self-limiting disease requiring continuous treatment (e.g., diabetes)
- 5 points → Non-self-limiting with complications (e.g., diabetic foot ulcers)
- 6 points → Diseases leading to permanent deformity or deterioration (e.g., paralytic stroke)

ÞÞÞ

After evaluating all five fields:
Add up the points from Intensity + Duration + Dreadfulness + Extent + Nature.
Example:

- Intensity: Moderate → 3 points
- Duration: 11 days to 1 month → 2 points
- Dreadfulness: Grade 1 pathological changes → 3 points
- Extent: Internal organ benign affection → 2 points
- Nature: Self-limiting with complications → 2 points

Disease Parameters subtotal = 3 + 2 + 3 + 2 + 2 = 12 points

ÞÞÞ

Important Points to Remember

- Minimum Disease Parameters subtotal = 5 (if all conditions are mild and new).
- Maximum Disease Parameters subtotal = 30 (if all conditions are severe and chronic).
- The Disease subtotal shows how serious, chronic, and deep the disease is in the patient.
- This subtotal is added directly to the Health Score to calculate the final HP Score.

ppp

How HP Score is Calculated

Step 1: Calculate the Health Sum

- First, you add together the subtotal points from these four sections:
- General Parameters subtotal (based on normal/abnormal function)
- Mental Generals subtotal (based on awareness, coping, productivity)
- Emotional Attributes subtotal (based on emotional health)
- History subtotal (based on past illness, family history, ongoing treatment, personal habits)

Formula: Health Sum = (General Parameters subtotal) + (Mental Generals subtotal) + (Emotional Attributes subtotal) + (History subtotal)

ᛒᛒᛒ

Step 2: Convert Health Sum into Health Score

The raw Health Sum is then converted into a Health Score according to a fixed rule:

- Health Sum 0–2 → Health Score 1
- Health Sum 3–4 → Health Score 2
- Health Sum 5–6 → Health Score 3
- Health Sum 7–8 → Health Score 4
- Health Sum 9–10 → Health Score 5
- Health Sum more than 10 → Health Score 6

Important:
The higher the Health Score, the worse the general health status of the patient.

ᛒᛒᛒ

Step 3: Calculate Disease Parameters Total

Next, you add together the five disease parameters:

- Intensity
- Duration
- Dreadfulness
- Extent
- Nature

Each parameter has a direct score from 1 to 6 based on severity.

Formula: Disease Parameters Total = (Intensity) + (Duration) + (Dreadfulness) + (Extent) + (Nature)

ᛒᛒᛒ

Step 4: Calculate HP Score

Finally, the HP Score is the sum of Health Score and Disease Parameters Total.

Formula: HP Score = Health Score + Disease Parameters Total

This HP Score determines the case level and management plan.

ᛒᛒᛒ

Step 5: Interpret the HP Score
Once the HP Score is calculated, it is classified into a Case Level:

- HP Score 6–10 → Level 1 (Simple case, symptom similarity is enough)
- HP Score 11–15 → Level 2 (Symptom similarity plus pathology consideration)
- HP Score 16–20 → Level 3 (Need to integrate symptom similarity + pathology + miasm analysis)
- HP Score 21–25 → Level 4 (Add surgical option if needed)
- HP Score 26–30 → Level 5 (Expert case, critical similimum selection)
- HP Score 31–36 → Level 6 (Palliative care needed)

Quick Summary of Full Flow:

- Calculate Health Sum
- Convert Health Sum to Health Score
- Calculate Disease Parameters Total
- Add both → HP Score
- Use HP Score to find Case Level and Plan Treatment

Curability Percent

- After you calculate the Health Score and the Disease Parameters Total, the system estimates how easily the disease can be cured.
- It compares the patient's general health status with the seriousness of the disease.
- If the patient's general health is good and the disease is not very advanced, the curability percent will be high.
- If the patient's general health is poor and the disease is severe, the curability percent will be low.
- If curability percent becomes more than 100, it is adjusted and capped at 100.
- If curability percent falls below 5 percent, it is declared as "<5%" meaning the case is nearly incurable.

In short:

- Higher curability percent means higher chances of cure.
- Lower curability percent means guarded or poor prognosis.

ppp

Disease Intensity

- Disease Intensity shows how deeply the disease has affected the body.
- It depends only on the Disease Parameters Total.
- If the total disease burden (intensity, duration, dreadfulness, extent, and nature) is high, the disease intensity will also be high.
- If the disease parameters are mild, the disease intensity will be low.

In short:

- Higher disease intensity means more serious or widespread disease.
- Lower disease intensity means a milder or limited disease condition.

ppp

Case Score

- Case Score tells how strong the patient's ability to overcome the disease is.
- It is calculated by checking how much healthy reserve remains compared to the disease burden.
- If the disease is mild, the case score will be high, meaning the body can easily respond to treatment.
- If the disease is heavy and complicated, the case score will be low, meaning the case will be slower to respond or difficult to manage.

In short:

- Higher case score means better recovery potential.
- Lower case score means weaker recovery ability.

Overall Simple Meaning

- Curability Percent tells about chances of cure.

- Disease Intensity tells about seriousness of the disease.
- Case Score tells about the body's ability to fight back.

THIRTY-FOUR
SCORING SCALES AND INTEGRATION

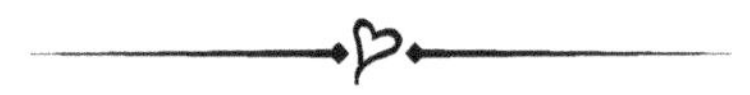

"The scoring scales of The Hidden Protocol are the foundation upon which objective analysis and effective decision-making rest. Each parameter is assigned a specific range that aligns with its clinical significance. This section outlines how these individual scores integrate into an aggregated system for assessing health, disease severity, and overall case complexity."

1. SCORING SCALES

1.1 General Parameters

Purpose: To assess physiological balance.

- Scale:

  - 0: Normal.
  - 0.5: Abnormal.

- Parameters Included:

  - Appetite, thirst, stool, urine, sweat, sleep.

1.2 Mental and Emotional Attributes

Purpose: To evaluate psychological and emotional contributions to health.

- Scale:

  - 0: Positive or functional.
  - 1: Moderate dysfunction.
  - 2: Severe dysfunction.

- *Parameters Included:*

  - Awareness, stress coping, productivity, emotional state, and mental contributions to illness.

1.3 Disease-Specific Parameters

Purpose: To determine the severity and progression of the disease.

- Scale:

  - Intensity: 1 (mild) to 6 (life-threatening).
  - Duration: 1 (<10 days) to 6 (>3 years).
  - Dreadfulness: 1 (reversible without medication) to 6 (irreversible).
  - Extent: 1 (single superficial organ) to 6 (multi-system/metastatic).
  - Nature: 1 (self-limiting) to 6 (requiring palliation).

1.4 Historical and Lifestyle Factors

Purpose: To identify predisposing and maintaining causes.

- Scale:

  - 0: No history or impact.
  - 1: Moderate history or impact.
  - 2: Significant history or impact.

- Parameters Included:

  - Past history, family history, treatment history, personal habits.

2. SCORE INTEGRATION

Scores from each parameter are combined into three primary indices:

- *2.1 Health Score*

  - Definition: Reflects the patient's overall health and physiological balance.
  - Calculation: Sum of all general and mental/emotional parameters.
  - Range:

    - 0 to 6: Optimal health.
    - 7 to 12: Moderate dysfunction.
    - 12: Significant dysfunction.

  - Interpretation:

    - Lower scores indicate better health; higher scores suggest areas needing attention.

- 2.2 Disease Score

  - Definition: Measures disease severity based on its intensity, duration, dreadfulness, extent, and nature.
  - Calculation: Sum of all disease-specific parameters.
  - Range:
  - 5 to 10: Mild cases.
  - 11 to 20: Moderate cases.
  - 21 to 30: Severe cases.
  - Interpretation:
  - Guides the practitioner on prognosis and treatment complexity.

- 2.3 Holistic Potential (HP) Score

  ○ Definition: Aggregates health and disease scores to determine the overall case complexity.

$$^{``}Calculation:$$
$$HP\ Score=Health\ Score+Disease\ Score^{"}$$

Range:

- **6 to 10: Level 1 (Simple Case).**
- **11 to 15: Level 2 (Careful Case).**
- **16 to 20: Level 3 (Cautious Case).**
- **21 to 25: Level 4 (Extra Care Case).**
- **26 to 30: Level 5 (Expert Case).**
- **31 to 36: Level 6 (Palliative Case).**

Interpretation:
Determines the treatment strategy, including the need for miasmatic analysis, surgical options, or palliative care.
3. Visual Representation

- 3.1 Graphs and Charts

  ○ Scores are best visualised through graphs to aid interpretation. Examples include:

    ▪ Curability Chart: Displays the patient's curability percentage.
    ▪ Disease Intensity Chart: Highlights the severity of disease parameters.
    ▪ Case Score Chart: Summarises the overall complexity.

- 3.2 Tabular Representation

  ○ Scores can also be tabulated for easier comparison and follow-ups.

4. Case Example
Patient Profile:
A 35-year-old female with chronic anxiety and hypothyroidism.
Scores:

- General Parameters: Appetite (0.5), Thirst (0), Sleep (0.5).
- Mental Attributes: Stress-coping (2), Productivity (1), Emotional State (1).
- Disease Parameters: Intensity (3), Duration (5), Extent (4).
- Historical Factors: Family History (2), Personal Habits (1).

Results:

- Health Score: 5.5.
- Disease Score: 15.
- HP Score: 20.

Case Level: Level 3 (Cautious Case).

"*The integration of scoring scales provides a robust framework for analysing cases. By systematically aggregating and interpreting these scores, homoeopathic practitioners can deliver evidence-based, personalised care.*"

THIRTY-FIVE

A SAMPLE REPORT

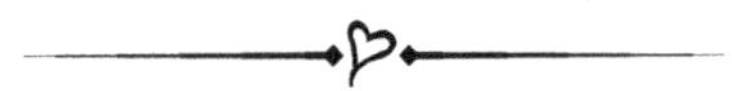

Name: GN
Age: 5 years
Sex: Female

Calculation Details

General Parameters:

- Appetite: Abnormal → 0.5 points
- Thirst: Normal → 0 points
- Stool: Abnormal → 0.5 points
- Urine: Normal → 0 points
- Sweat: Abnormal → 0.5 points
- Sleep: Abnormal → 0.5 points
- Menses: Not applicable → 0 points

Subtotal from General Parameters = 2 points.

Mental Generals:

- Awareness of Abilities: Well aware → 0 points
- Stress Coping Level: Somewhat coped → 1 point
- Productivity and Fruitfulness: Moderate → 1 point

Subtotal from Mental Generals = 2 points.

Emotional Attributes:

- Mental Attributes Contributing to Illness: Yes → 2 points
- Level on Emotional Scale: Moderate negative emotions → 1 point

Subtotal from Emotional Attributes = 3 points.

History:

- Past History: Very Strong → 2 points
- Family History: Moderate → 1 point
- Treatment History: No History → 0 points
- Personal History: Moderate → 1 point

Subtotal from History = 4 points.

Total Health Sum: 2 (General Parameters) + 2 (Mental Generals) + 3 (Emotional Attributes) + 4 (History) = 11 points.

Conversion to Health Score:

- Health Sum of 11 converts to Health Score 6 (as per Hidden Protocol).
- Health Score = 6.

Disease Parameters:

- Intensity: Moderate → 3 points
- Duration: 11 days to 1 month → 2 points
- Dreadfulness: Grade 1 pathological changes → 3 points
- Extent: Internal organ benign affection → 2 points
- Nature: Self-limiting with complications → 2 points

Subtotal from Disease Parameters = 12 points.

HP Score Calculation:

HP Score = Health Score + Disease Parameters Total

HP Score = 6 + 12 = 18

HP Level Interpretation:

- HP Score 16 to 20 falls under Level 3.

Interpretation:
Case requires careful integration of symptom similarity, pathology evaluation, and miasmatic analysis.
Curability Percent:

- Calculated curability percent is less than 5%.

Interpretation: *Prognosis guarded; case tending toward incurability unless extraordinary response occurs.*
Disease Intensity:

- Disease intensity is approximately 33.33%.

Case Score:

- Case score is approximately 66.67%.

Final Summary for GN

Health Score: 6
    Disease Parameter Total: 12
    HP Score: 18
    HP Level: Level 3
    Curability Percent: Less than 5%
    Disease Intensity: 33.33%
    Case Score: 66.67%

Clinical Interpretation for GN

The low curability rate (less than 5%) combined with a disease intensity of 33.33% indicates that the child is constitutionally weak.

This weakness reflects an inherent disturbance in the child's biological balance, likely due to deep-seated miasmatic influences.

Therefore, the therapeutic approach must focus on:

- Administering appropriate anti-miasmatic remedies,
- Aiming to gradually strengthen the constitutional vitality,
- Restoring systemic balance at the genetic and dynamic levels.

Important Note:

- Even after improvement, the child's susceptibility to disease will remain higher compared to a constitutionally stronger individual.
- Thus, long-term follow-up and periodic constitutional support will be necessary to maintain health stability and prevent recurrence.

THIRTY-SIX

KEY INSIGHTS FROM DR. P. RADHAKRISHNAN'S EXPERIENCE

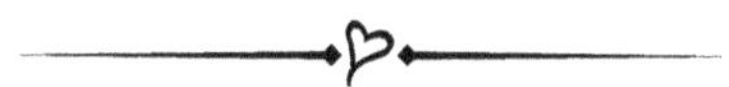

Adaptability

""The protocol is not rigid; it breathes with the needs of each patient.""

Precision and Compassion:

""A good homoeopath is precise, but a great one balances precision with empathy.""

Confidence in Complexity:

""The Hidden Protocol empowers practitioners to face even the gravest cases with unwavering confidence.""

A Compass for Every Practitioner

"The Hidden Protocol is not just a tool; it's a compass for homoeopaths. Whether you're managing a simple fever or a life-threatening disease, this scoring system guides you towards clarity, precision, and compassion. It standardises treatment plans without diluting the essence of individualisation—a true revolution in homoeopathic care."

A Gift to Homoeopaths Worldwide

Dr P. Nidheesh, inspired by his father's clinical brilliance, developed these indices to make the art of homoeopathy more scientific, standardised, and universally applicable. This tool is not just a system; it is a gift to the homoeopathic community, empowering practitioners to treat patients with precision and confidence.

"The Hidden Protocol transforms subjective intuition into objective clarity, guiding homoeopaths to the right treatment every time."
– Dr P. Nidheesh

A Revolution In Homoeopathic Treatment

Homoeopathy, a profound science of healing, has always thrived on individualisation and precision. However, the complexity of integrating subjective symptoms, pathology, and miasmatic influences often makes treatment planning a daunting task. To bridge this gap, The Hidden Protocol emerges as a groundbreaking tool—a meticulously crafted scoring system designed to standardise and streamline the plan of treatment while maintaining the essence of homoeopathy.

This protocol is the culmination of decades of clinical expertise and visionary thinking by Dr P. Radhakrishnan, a legend in homoeopathy since 1976. With over 47 years of experience, he has treated countless patients across a spectrum of conditions, ranging from the mildest to the most severe, including life-threatening diseases. His unparalleled insight into the human body and mind, honed through lakhs of consultations, has been channelled into creating this blessed tool—a guiding light for homoeopaths worldwide.

Uniqueness Of The Hidden Protocol

The Hidden Protocol stands apart as a revolutionary advancement in homoeopathy due to its blend of tradition and modernity. Its uniqueness lies in the following key features:

Systematic Approach:

- Converts subjective case elements into objective scores, ensuring clarity and precision in case evaluation.

Comprehensive Coverage:

- Integrates general, mental, emotional, and disease-specific parameters, making it a holistic diagnostic tool.

Guided Treatment Plan:

- Generates a clear, actionable plan of treatment based on the scoring system, removing ambiguities and reducing errors.

Tailored for Individualisation:

- Maintains the core principle of homoeopathy by allowing for nuanced interpretations of each patient's unique constitution.

Standardisation:

- Offers a standardised framework for treatment planning, ensuring consistency in outcomes across practices and practitioners.

Prognostic Insights:

- Provides a reliable estimation of curability and treatment duration, empowering homoeopaths to set realistic expectations for their patients.

Versatile Application:

- Can be adapted to various specialisations, including chronic diseases, acute care, and integrative medicine.

Tech-Enabled:

- Ready for integration with digital tools, enhancing accessibility and ease of use in modern clinical settings.

A Visionary Tool By Dr P. Radhakrishnan

Dr P. Radhakrishnan's philosophy is rooted in the belief that "a well-informed homoeopath is empowered to treat the gravest of conditions with confidence." His experience of witnessing the transformative power of homoeopathy in countless lives inspired him to develop this protocol as a blessing for practitioners.

> "*The Hidden Protocol isn't just a tool; it is a trusted companion for every homoeopath. It guides, enlightens, and empowers the practitioner to deliver the best possible care, ensuring that no case, however challenging, is beyond reach.*"
> *– Dr P. Radhakrishnan*

Having encountered lakhs of cases, ranging from mild fevers to life-threatening cancers, Dr Radhakrishnan understands the importance of systematic treatment planning. The Hidden Protocol encapsulates his lifetime of learning, offering every homoeopath the ability to think and act with the precision of decades of experience.

The Major Speciality: A Blessed Tool For Standardising Treatment

The most remarkable aspect of The Hidden Protocol is its ability to standardise treatment plans without compromising the individualisation central to homoeopathy. By providing practitioners with a structured framework, this tool ensures:

Clarity in Decision-Making:

- Practitioners know exactly how to proceed with treatment, step-by-step.

Confidence in Severe Cases:

- The protocol offers reliable guidance, even in the most complex and severe cases.

Efficiency in Practice:

- Reduces the cognitive load on practitioners, enabling them to focus on the art of healing.

Consistency Across Practices:

- Sets a benchmark for quality care, ensuring uniformity in outcomes regardless of the practitioner.

Enhanced Patient Trust:

- Patients feel reassured by the transparency and systematic approach to their treatment.